Why this is the ultimate diet...

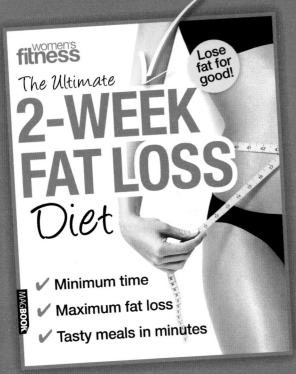

wf It will make your body a fat-burning machine

wf It will shrink your fat cells

Reach your fat loss goal

wf It's super easy to follow and stick to

wf It will help you shed fat today and every day until you reach your fat loss goal

So what are you waiting for...?

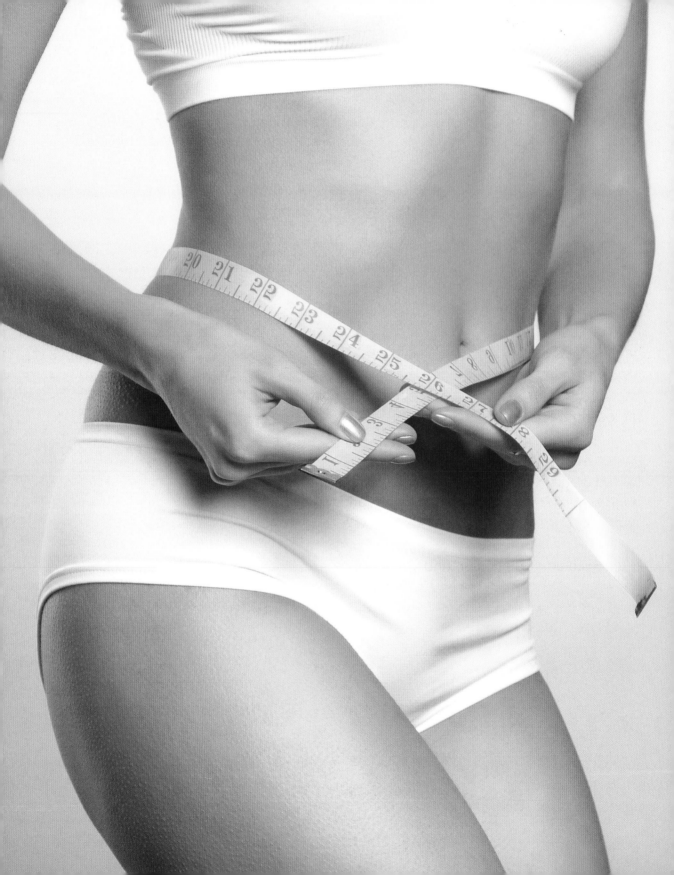

Editor's note

Guess what? We've discovered the *real* secrets to quick, healthy and long-lasting fat loss. Yes, really! So, we've decided to share them with you in *The Ultimate 2-Week Fat Loss Diet*. Not only will this book help you to shed fat for good, it actually shrinks your fat cells, too.

First up, we bring you the most up-to-the minute research into fat-burning techniques (from page 13), whether it's eating more pink seafood or upping your omega-3. Bursting with simple tips and tricks, this guide will put your fat loss in the fast lane, forever!

Armed with your new fat-shrinking know-how, you're then ready to start the 2-week diet (from page 77). Forget hunger – think tasty, delicious and filling foods that encourage your fat loss while staving off cravings.

It really couldn't be easier, and you'll notice the results in just two weeks. So read on to discover how to burn fat the easy way!

Joanna

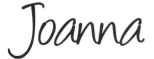

women's fitness

Editor Joanna Knight
Sub-Editor Charlotte Cox
Art Director Matt Reynolds
Author Fiona Kirk
Photography StockFood, Shutterstock
Cover Shutterstock

Digital Production Manager Nicky Baker
MagBook Publisher Dharmesh Mistry
Operations Director Robin Ryan
Advertising Manager Katie Wood
MD of Advertising Julian Lloyd-Evans
Newstrade Director David Barker
Chief Operating Officer Brett Reynolds
Group Finance Director Ian Leggett
Chief Executive James Tye
Chairman Felix Dennis

MAGBOOK

The MagBook brand is a trademark of Dennis Publishing Ltd. 30 Cleveland St, London W1T 4JD. Company registered in England. All material © Dennis Publishing Ltd, licensed by Felden 2011, and may not be reproduced in whole or part without the consent of the publishers. *The Ultimate 2-Week Fat Loss Diet* ISBN 1781060053.

Licensing & Syndication
To license this product please contact Hannah Heagney on +44 (0) 20 7907 6134 or email hannah_heagney@dennis.co.uk
To syndicate content from this product please contact Anj Dosaj Halai on +44 (0) 20 7907 6132 or email anj_dosaj-halai@dennis.co.uk

Liability
While every care was taken during the production of this MagBook, the publishers cannot be held responsible for the accuracy of the information or any consequence arising from it. Dennis Publishing takes no responsibility for the companies advertising in this MagBook. The paper used within this MagBook is produced from sustainable fibre, manufactured by mills with a valid chain of custody. Printed at BGPrint Ltd.

Always check with your GP before starting a diet or exercise programme, especially if you are pregnant, breast feeding or have been inactive for a long time. Those with a history of high blood pressure or heart disease should obtain medical clearance before undertaking any activity.

Contents

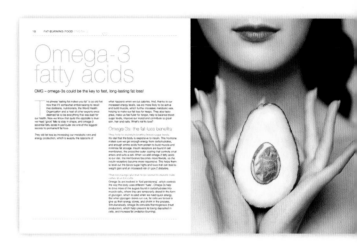

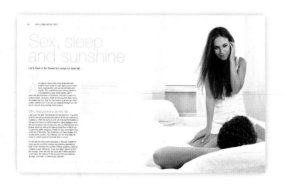

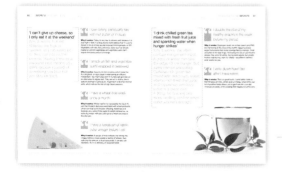

2-week action plan

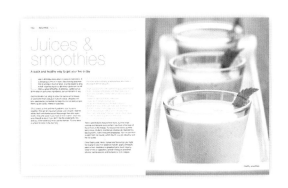

Fat-burning recipes

Enjoy delicious meals at breakfast, lunch and dinner

Quick-fix rescue plan

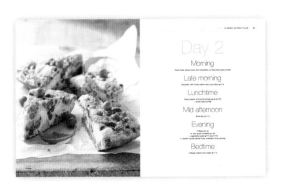

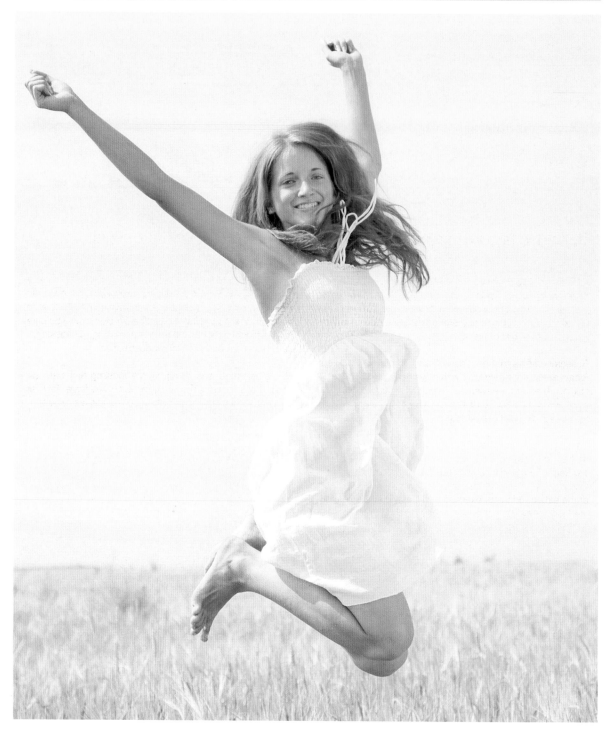

The secret to success

Forget the fads and say no-no to the yo-yo, this is a diet that really works

Should we accept that the only way to shed fat for good is by slow, dragged-out dieting? No way! If we put our minds to it, we can change our eating habits and see some great results in just a matter of weeks.

Research shows that between 85 and 95 per cent of dieters regain any weight they lose within five years and, worse still, some end up heavier than when they started. But what about the 5 to 15 per cent who reach their goal and maintain their initial weight loss?

After months of interviewing many people of both sexes and all ages, we've made a rather surprising discovery: 63 per cent of the successful dieters found a *quick* diet that worked! Their initial fat loss spurred them into keeping some of the eating, drinking, exercise and lifestyle strategies for the long-term; and not only did they reach their fat-loss goal, they maintained it.

It's quick, but not quick fix!

This book presents a diet that will give you maximum fat loss with maximum nourishment in minimum time. It is not a crash diet, it does not restrict calories or leave you short of nutritional goodness, it is not depressing, distressing, demotivating, demoralising or destructive.

It is a balanced, energising, mood-boosting two-week diet that brings together the latest research into faster fat loss with some inspiring tips from successful dieters. You'll be tucking into:

– foods that encourage fat loss
– foods that turn up the fat-burning mechanism
– foods that delay hunger and conquer cravings
– foods that make you feel good
– foods that fire up your sex drive
– foods that help you sleep

You'll also learn when and how to exercise to achieve maximum fat loss in minimum time. It's sure to send your results into overdrive!

Why does it work?

Women have around 34 billion fat cells and men have around 25 billion. When we gain fat, we are not gaining new fat cells, we are merely expanding the ones we already have. They can grow to five times their size, so to lose fat we have to get them to shrink – and stay shrunk! There are certain elements that can give them a boost and that's what we're going to concentrate on. Let the fat burning begin...

Real women's secrets to success

Bin the diet drinks

'I always had a can of Diet Coke nearby and believed that because it was 'diet' it didn't add calories to my day. I learned that these supposedly negative calories did nothing to stem my dependence on sugar. So, I replaced most of them with fresh fruit juices mixed 50/50 with sparkling water, and I couldn't believe the reduction in my sugar cravings! I now understand that it was my need for sugar that had foiled every attempt at fat loss over many years.'

Still enjoy pasta

'I love pasta and pasta loves me! It sits way too comfortably on my hips and thighs. After a hard day at the office, I loved a comforting bowl of Bolognese. I learned that I was enjoying my favourite Italian export at the wrong time of the day. Now, if I want pasta, I have it at lunchtime when I need the immediate energy it provides to get me through the day.'

Eat fish to beat hunger

'I never liked fish – all those heads, bones and eyes staring up at me were enough to turn my stomach. But the diet I was trying to follow championed the power of omega-3 fatty acids to stem hunger pangs. I persevered and found a man behind the fish counter in my local supermarket who removed the heads and bones and suggested ways to cook it. Now I eat fish at least four times a week.'

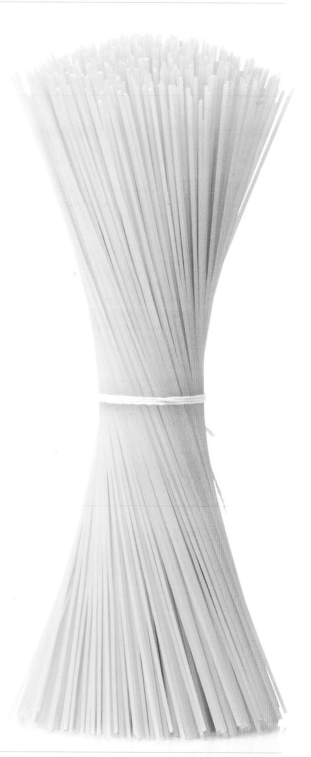

Picture it

'Loads of diets I had been on encouraged me to write a food diary. But I always lied. Yes, I'd mentioned the chocolate biscuit I had with my afternoon cup of tea... I would just forget to mention that it wasn't just one, it was four! One diet that I came across suggested that I bin the pen and paper and use my mobile phone to record everything I eat in a day in photo form. Revealing or what? I couldn't believe how much junk I managed to fit into a day. I followed the diet to the letter and within a couple of days I loved looking at pictures of the colourful health-giving foods that were now part of my day.'

Steam to be healthy

'The reason I maintained my weight loss is because I learned how to steam food. I had never steamed food before, so it was a new experience and has been a real life-changer. I bought a set of steam baskets and found lots of recipes on the internet for preparing really quick, healthy, tasty meals. The frying pan has been relegated to the back of the cupboard.'

Get your five-a-day

'I always struggled to meet my five-a-day fruit and veg target. However, I realised that if I could find ways to make it more exciting I might be onto a winner. Fruits were fairly easy to include, but vegetables were still a struggle; so I focused on the five vegetables that I really liked and researched lots of different ways to prepare them (and had big portions to fill me up). I reached my target weight after six weeks and haven't put on a pound since. My diet is now a lot more colourful – and anything but dull.'

Find alternatives

'I shared a flat with a Chinese girl and the first thing I noticed was that when we went shopping, almost no dairy products hit her trolley. This made me realise just how much cows' milk, butter and cheese were involved in my daily diet. My flatmate introduced me to a few delicious alternatives, particularly nut and seed oils and butters and soya milk, and my weight started to plummet only 10 days after making the changes. I now eat the Asian way most days and, while I still relish every bite of a takeaway four-cheese pizza, it has become an occasional treat rather than a weekly must-have.'

Bounce your way slim

'I've always hated exercise, while Googling 'fast fat loss,' I discovered rebounding (exercise using a mini trampoline) and I reckoned it was worth a try. What can I say? I became obsessed with that little trampoline and instead of slobbing on the couch throughout an entire movie, I started to bounce my way through half of it! Alongside a diet that includes lots of healthy stuff but still allows me to have lots of good nights out with my friends, it really works. After six months I am now very lean and, while I still hate exercise, me and my mini trampoline are not just flirting with each other, we are in a long-term relationship!'

Freeze it

'It seems that every diet I have ever tried involved way too much shopping. All the nutrients that are important for fat loss appear to be richest in fresh foods, but after the first few days of struggling to find the time to shop fresh, I always returned to ready-made chilled foods. When I spotted a diet on the internet that promised weight loss by eating foods from the freezer, I learned that frozen fruits and vegetables are packed with almost as much nutritional punch as their fresh counterparts (sometimes more). If you have a few bags in the freezer you can create soups and smoothies, super-fast! I now always have at least six bags of frozen fruits and vegetables in the freezer and no longer have a weight problem.'

Get seedy

'I went on a diet that recommended linseed to keep hunger at bay. A bit more reading made me realise that the good fats in linseed would fill me up and keep my blood sugar balanced for longer. I started sprinkling the seeds on my salads, drizzling the oil on my soups and vegetables and snacking on seed bars that included them. I have lost more than two stone, and I have linseeds to thank.'

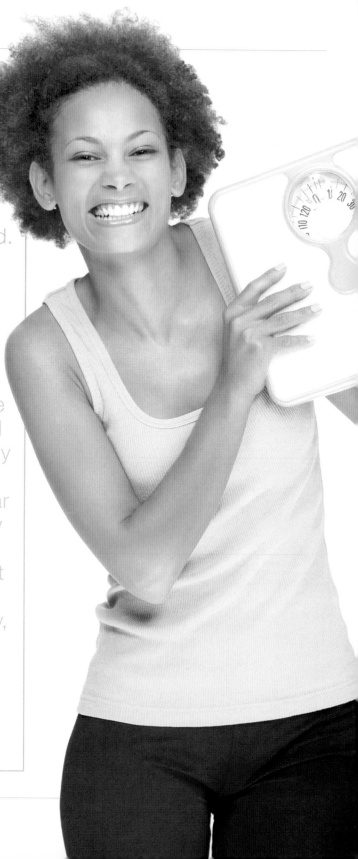

Bin the scales

'I binned the scales and used the waistband method. Instead of watching a little needle waver frustratingly from right to left every morning, I put on a pair of jeans that were too tight on me. After two weeks of dieting, I could get a couple of thumbs between me and the waistband and this really inspired me to keep going. I have always been a regular snacker as I was constantly hungry, but instead of the crisps and salty snacks that were my downfall, I started to keep a few of the healthy, filling snacks in my desk drawer. Small changes can reap big rewards, as the fact that I now feel great in my skinny jeans shows!'

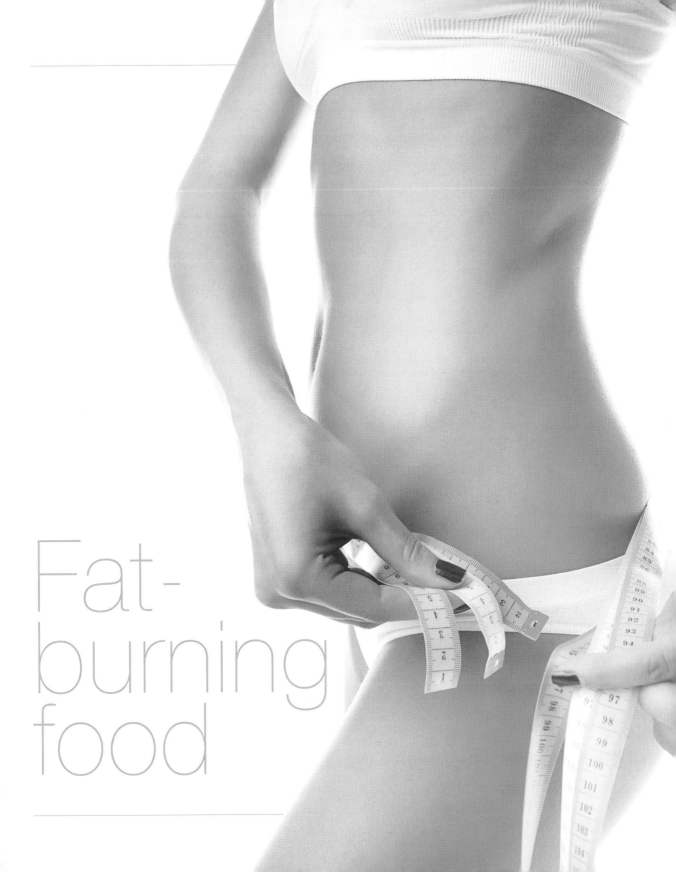

Fat-
burning
food

Calcium

It's not just good for our bones, it gets us gorgeous bodies, too!

We all know of the importance of calcium in our diet to build and maintain strong bones and teeth. But how much have you heard about its fat-busting properties? Recent research reveals that this bone strengthener may also be a fat blaster!

A growing body of evidence indicates that a diet rich in calcium allows us to burn more calories per day. There is also some evidence that when calcium levels in the body are low the brain detects this and stimulates feelings of hunger, causing us to eat more. Conversely, medium to high levels send signals to the brain communicating that we are full, suppressing the desire to eat more.

Calcium intake:
– LOW: less than 600mg per day
– MEDIUM: 600-1,000mg per day
– HIGH: 1,000mg plus per day

It has also been suggested that increasing calcium in the diet may reduce the transportation of fat from the intestines into the bloodstream. The calcium binds with bile acids to increase the amount of fat we excrete through the bowel, so instead of storing it, we lose it!

Too much milk?

Milk is a valuable source of calcium up until about the age of 18, when we are still growing. Thereafter we can have too much of a good thing. Milk with our morning cereals, milk in our coffee and tea, butter on our toast, cream in our cakes, cheese in our sandwiches and snacks, ice cream at the movies...the list goes on.

The protein in milk can acidify the blood, and our bodies are forced to extract calcium from our bones to counteract this. Furthermore, milk fat can contribute to inflammation within the body and possible intolerance to lactose, the sugar in milk products. To prevent this debilitating condition while still reaping the calcium benefits, less is definitely more on the dairy front. *The Ultimate 2-Week Fat Loss Diet* achieves this by only including yoghurt, which actually improves lactose absorption thanks to its active live cultures, and certain cheeses that fall into the low lactose category.

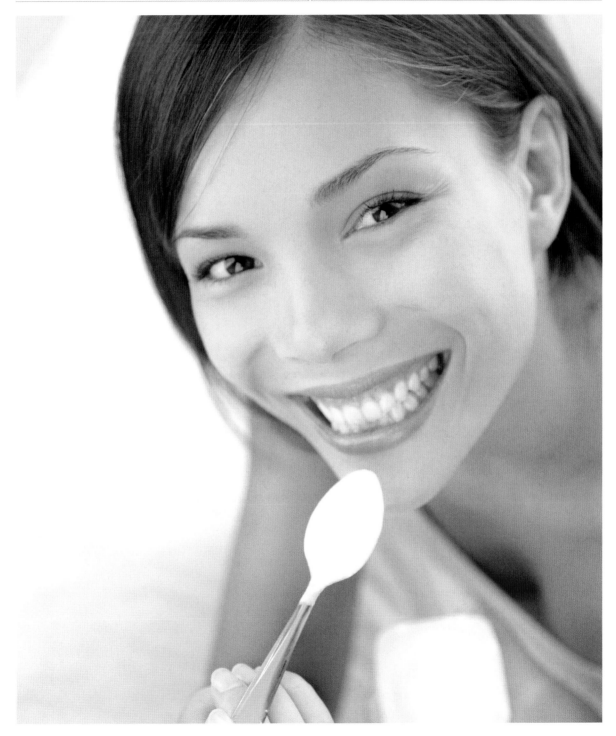

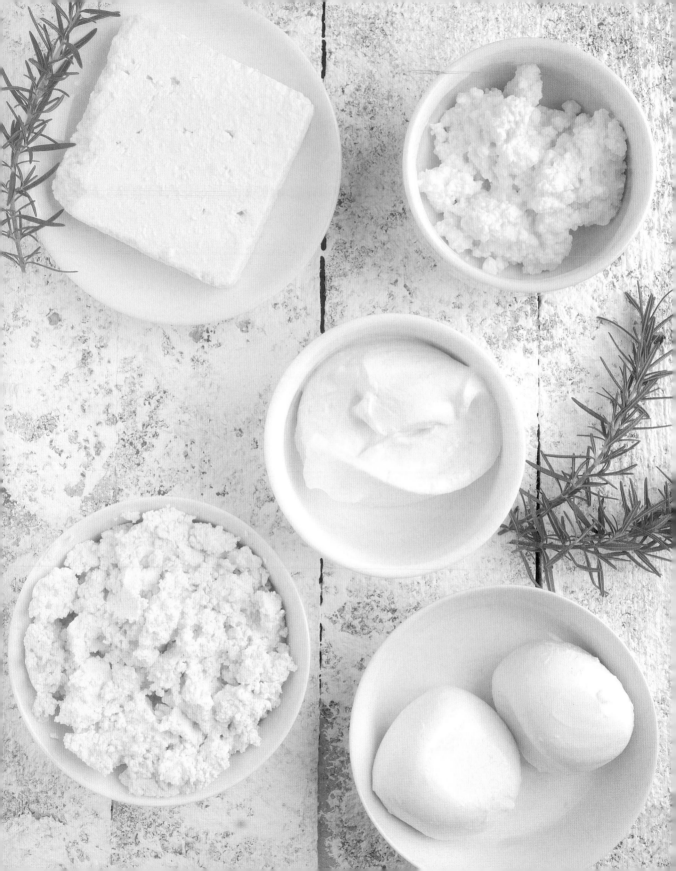

The calcium-packed alternatives

The fossilised bones of our earliest ancestors indicate that they ingested around twice as much calcium daily as we do now, and they were lean – very lean. But for them, dairy was a complete unknown (animals simply didn't hang around long enough to be milked). So what did they eat?

To build and maintain strong bones we need not only calcium but also magnesium, vitamin D, boron, manganese, molybdenum, vitamin K, zinc, copper, vitamin B6 and the omega-3 and omega-6 fatty acids. The diet of our early ancestors comprised of red meat and birds (and they ate every part of the animal including the organs), fish and shellfish (including the bones and heads, which are very rich in calcium), root vegetables, sea vegetables, green leafy plants and birds' eggs (including the shells – another great source of calcium). This provided them with good levels of all of the above nutrients. And, of course, their active lifestyle further enhanced bone growth and kept them lean.

While we're not suggesting that you start crunching on eggshells and gnawing at bones, you will note that tinned salmon, sardines and anchovies feature regularly because they offer an ideal opportunity to get some calcium-rich bones into your day!

Calcium-rich foods in the 2-week diet
- Calcium-enriched soya milk
- Dried herbs
- Dried/tinned beans
- Edamame beans
- Feta cheese
- Fresh/frozen broccoli
- Fresh/frozen rhubarb
- Fresh/frozen spinach
- Fresh nuts and their oils and butters
- Fresh seeds and their oils and butters
- Fresh/tinned anchovies
- Fresh/tinned sardines
- Goats' cheese
- Kale
- Low fat natural cottage cheese
- Pak choy
- Parmesan cheese
- Regular tofu (smoked and unsmoked)
- Ricotta cheese
- Silken tofu
- Swiss cheese (with holes)
- Tinned salmon
- Total 0% Greek yoghurt
- Watercress

Did you know?
Increasing our consumption of cows' milk products to ensure good levels of calcium in our diet may be a bit of a red herring

Omega-3 fatty acids

OMG – omega-3s could be the key to fast, long-lasting fat loss!

The phrase 'eating fat makes you fat' is so old hat now that it's somewhat embarrassing to recall that dietitians, nutritionists, the World Health Organisation and a host of other experts once deemed fat to be everything that was bad for our health. Now we know that quite the opposite is true: we need 'good' fats to stay in shape, and omega-3 essential fatty acids in particular are one of the biggest secrets to permanent fat loss.

They aid fat loss by increasing our metabolic rate and energy production, which is exactly the opposite of what happens when we cut calories. And, thanks to our increased energy levels, we are more likely to be active and build muscle, which further increases metabolic rate, helping to make our fat loss for keeps. They also taste great, make us feel fuller for longer, help to balance blood sugar levels, improve our mood and contribute to great skin, hair and nails. What's not to love?

Omega-3s: the fat-loss benefits

They help to maintain healthy blood sugar levels

It's vital that the body is responsive to insulin. This hormone makes sure we get enough energy from carbohydrates, and enough amino acids from protein to build muscle and minimise fat storage. Insulin receptors are found in cell membranes, the protective outer coating that controls what enters and exits a cell. When we add omega-3 fatty acids to our diet, the membranes becomes more flexible, so the insulin receptors become more responsive. This helps them to level out the blood sugar highs and lows that can lead to weight gain and an increased risk of type 2 diabetes.

They encourage glucose to be stored in muscle cells rather than fat cells

Omega-3s are involved in 'fuel partitioning', which controls the way the body uses different 'fuels'. Omega-3s help to drive more of the sugars found in carbohydrates into muscle cells, where they are temporarily stored in the form of glycogen, which is used when we need quick energy. But when glycogen stores run out, fat cells are forced to give up their energy stores, and shrink in the process. Simultaneously, omega-3s stimulate thermogenesis (heat production), which helps prevent fat being deposited in cells, and increase fat oxidation (burning).

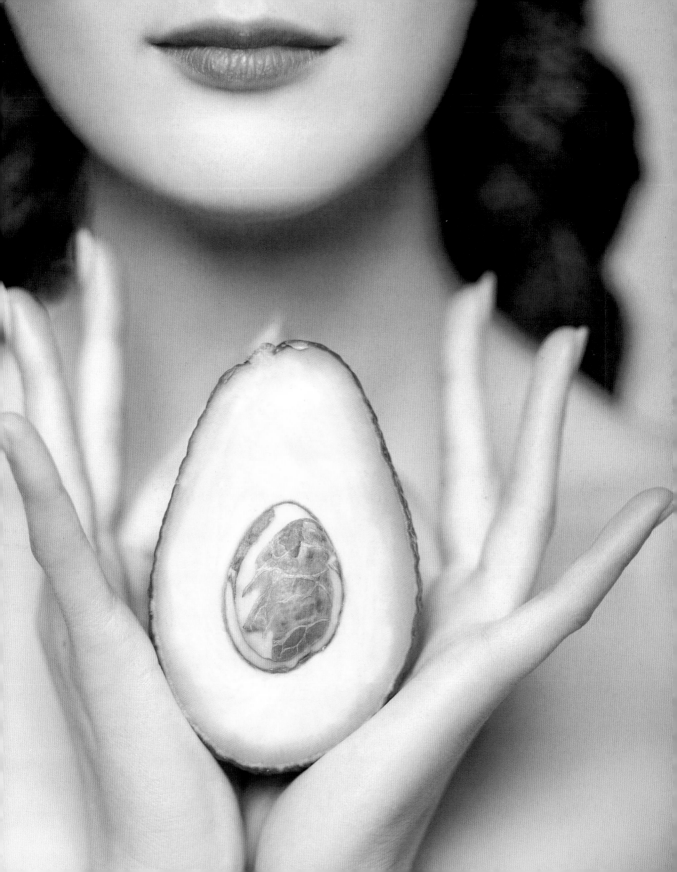

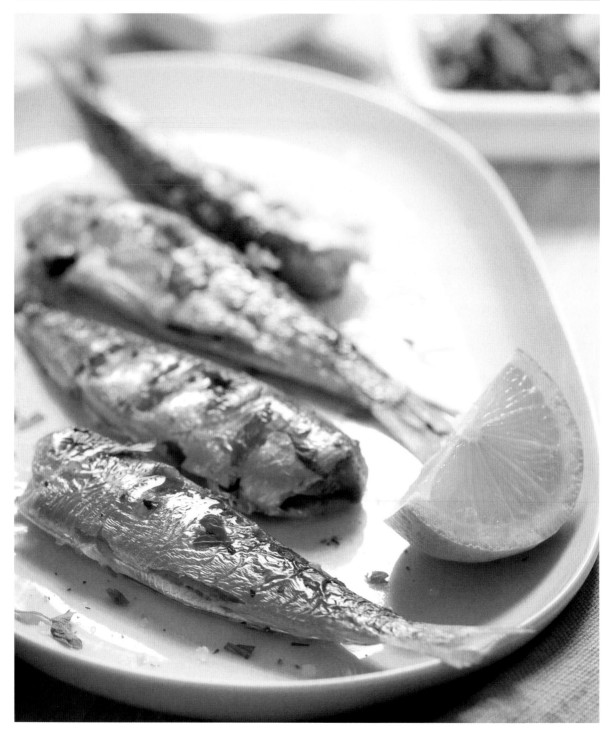

Thermogenesis is the production of heat within the body, where mitochondria in fat and muscle cells produce heat instead of energy. Body temperature rises, fat is used for energy and calories are burned. Research suggests that omega-3s may be able to influence genes that control how we burn fat. This may be due to a steroid-like substance in our bodies which, when bound to omega-3s, can switch on genes that burn fat. Omega-3s may also switch on a protein that aids energy metabolism, resulting in more energy being dissipated as heat and decreasing stored fat.

They inhibit the storage of calories as fat

It is important to remember that our species is programmed to survive, and this involves storing energy as fat. An efficient energy source, fat provides 9kcals of energy per gram, whereas carbohydrates and protein only provide 4kcals. Storing fat was vital to our ancestors as an insurance against times of starvation, so the body stored as much as possible when food was available, and the metabolic rate slowed down to preserve energy stores when food was scarce. This process has been referred to as catch-up fat storage after calorie restriction.

Food is now plentiful and many of us eat what we want, when we want, and this catch-up fat storage has become the enemy in the fat-loss game. The body stores energy as fat for lean times ahead, totally unaware that these are unlikely to occur. This is why very low-calorie diets invariably result in short term weight loss followed by weight gain. The catch-up fat storage shifts into top gear!

A system of enzymes (catalysts that speed up chemical reactions) called fatty acid synthase is particularly proficient at storing calories as fat. There is growing interest in the role omega-3s may have in reducing its power, thus increasing the likelihood of fat being burned rather than stored. Studies also suggest that omega-3s may be able to boost the production of certain enzymes involved in fatty acid oxidation, which helps transport fats into the mitochondria (energy factories) of the cells for burning as energy.

Omega 3-rich foods included in the 2-week diet:
— Avocado
— Avocado oil
— Dried and tinned chickpeas
— Dried and tinned kidney beans
— Eggs
— Fresh and frozen peas
— Fresh and smoked mackerel
— Fresh and tinned anchovies
— Fresh and tinned sardines
— Fresh and tinned tuna
— Hemp seeds
— Hemp seed oil
— Linseeds
— Linseed oil
— Rainbow trout
— Walnuts
— Walnut oil

Carbohydrates

Exciting news, everyone! Certain carbs can actually *burn* fat. Yes, really!

They've been demonised by diet after diet – but carbs don't deserve the bad wrap. In fact, the latest nutrient causing all the weight-loss buzz is *fermentable* carbohydrates. They don't add too much to our daily calorie intake, yet this wonder-nutrient promotes bowel regularity, reduces the chances of the pancreas getting overtired from keeping blood sugar levels constant and is associated with less fat storage after a meal. Wow!

So how does it work?

In essence, it's all about starch. The type of starch in carbohydrates predicts how quickly they will be broken down into smaller glucose molecules by the digestive enzymes in the mouth, the stomach and the small intestine. The quicker they are broken down, the quicker they are absorbed into the bloodstream and delivered to the liver, where they are either stored for later use or ferried off to body cells to create energy.

The starch in digestible carbohydrates can be divided into two groups: rapidly digestible starch (digested within 20 minutes), and slowly digestible starch (digested somewhere between 20 minutes and two hours).

Rapidly digested starch (RDS) is easily broken down and causes blood glucose to rise quickly, but then drop swiftly, too. This spike drives up the production of insulin, which tells the body to make and store fat. Foods rich in RDS include potatoes, processed foods made with white flour (bread and rolls, pastries, cakes, biscuits etc) and many breakfast cereals.

Non-digestible (fermentable) carbohydrates are a different breed, and are so called because they contain resistant starch (RS). They are largely resistant to being broken down into glucose molecules and absorbed into the bloodstream – instead they carry on down to the colon, where they go through a fermentation process that produces short chain fatty acids (SCFAs). These have a number of health benefits, detailed overleaf.

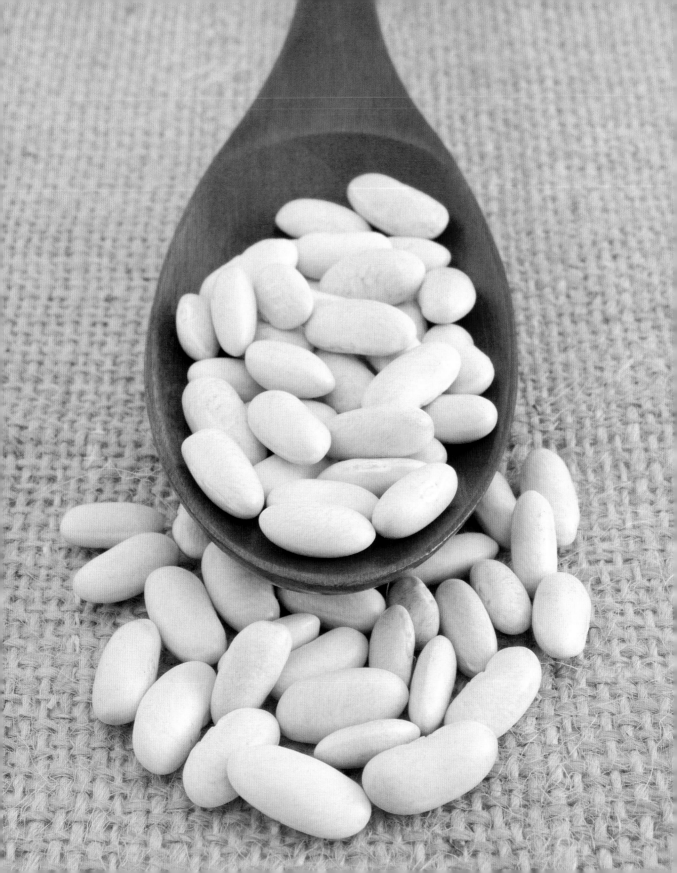

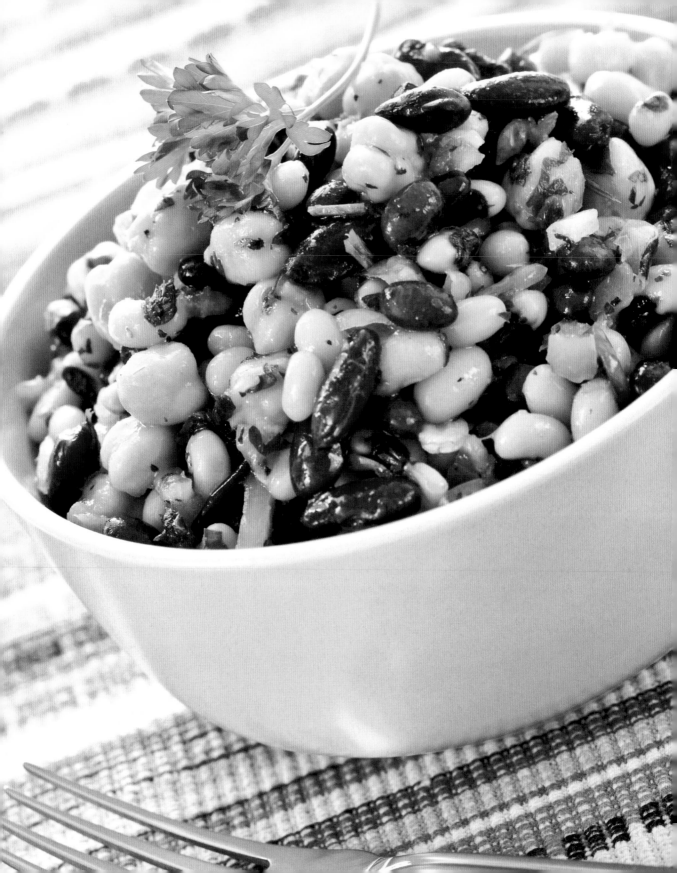

Health benefits of SCFAs:

Short chain fatty acids can boost our bodies in a number of ways:

— They protect colon cells, and are associated with preventing genetic damage that can lead to cancer.
— They increase mineral absorption, particularly that of calcium and magnesium. These nutrients are important for heart and bone health.
— They feed our healthy bacteria, which means that the growth of unhealthy bacteria and their toxic by-products is suppressed.

But how do fermentable carbs burn fat?

Resistant starch has little effect on blood glucose levels and doesn't drive up the production of insulin, which means the body is not encouraged to make or store fat. Non-digestible carbs have also been shown to encourage fat loss in a number of ways:

— They help to slow down the pace at which digestible carbohydrates get broken down, thereby reducing the counterproductive blood sugar highs and lows that cause us to reach for yet more starchy carbohydrates.
— They keep us feeling fuller for longer, so we eat less.
— They increase the absorption of calcium, which is linked to reducing fat storage.
— They promote bowel regularity. Constipation is no friend when fat loss is desired.
— They encourage a phenomenon known as 'second meal effect', where the insulin response is controlled not just straight after eating, but for hours afterwards, resulting in less fat storage.

Fermentable carbohydrates included in the 2-week diet:
— Barley
— Beans
— Brown rice
— Corn
— Lentils
— Millet
— Oats
— Split peas

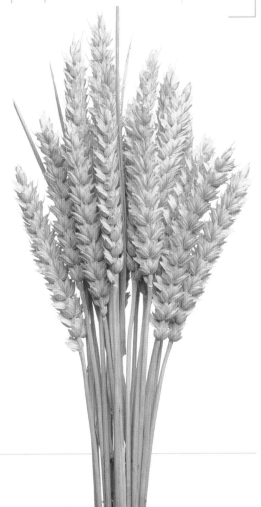

Spices

Want to set your fat-loss on fire? Spice up your diet to sizzle away the calories!

The traditional idea that fat cells are simply a storage depot for energy has now been proven wrong, wrong wrong. Fat cells are actually very active and produce hormones that trigger metabolic processes in different parts of the body.

The hormones produced by fat include oestradiol, a precursor to oestrogen, which controls reproduction; leptin, which controls the appetite by binding to receptors in the brain, telling us when we are full; and adiponectin, which controls blood sugar levels.

Key term: free radical

A free radical is an atom that has lost an electron from its outer orbit and becomes unstable. In a desperate bid to restore its stability, it randomly steals an electron from another atom, which in turn becomes unstable and is forced to go on the hunt. This domino effect means that thousands of free radical reactions can occur in seconds, threatening both the outer membranes of body cells and their DNA, which can alter the way they behave.

However, research has also revealed that fatty tissue produces inflammatory chemicals. Inflammation is a vital process in the body; it is the body's natural response to harmful substances, where dead or dying tissue is disposed and healing is promoted. Without it, wounds would not heal and disease could not be reversed.

Acute inflammation occurs when we are injured – the response is rapid, the duration is short and the process is efficient. However, chronic (ongoing) inflammation is a different story. This is when the healing process goes into overdrive and damaging free radicals (see left) are formed.

Overeating = inflammation

When we overeat, fat cells expand and if they are regularly over-stuffed (particularly those around the midriff) inflammatory chemicals leap into action and interfere with our weight-controlling hormones. As a result, we become less sensitive to signals telling us we're full, so we eat more and our insulin response is dulled. This causes episodes of hypoglycaemia (low blood sugar) that prompt us to reach for more food to counteract the tiredness, fuzzy brain, irritability and low mood that go with the territory.

Ballooning fat cells caused by overeating aren't the only reason that inflammatory chemicals are stimulated. Another major cause is what we actually eat. The altered fats and added sugars found in fried, fast, processed and junk foods are the chief culprits here.

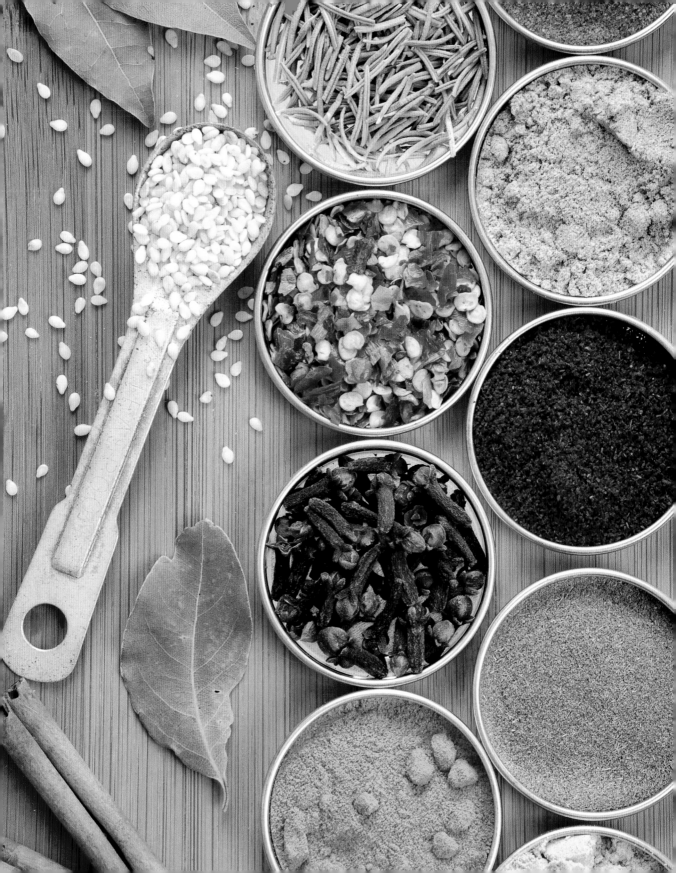

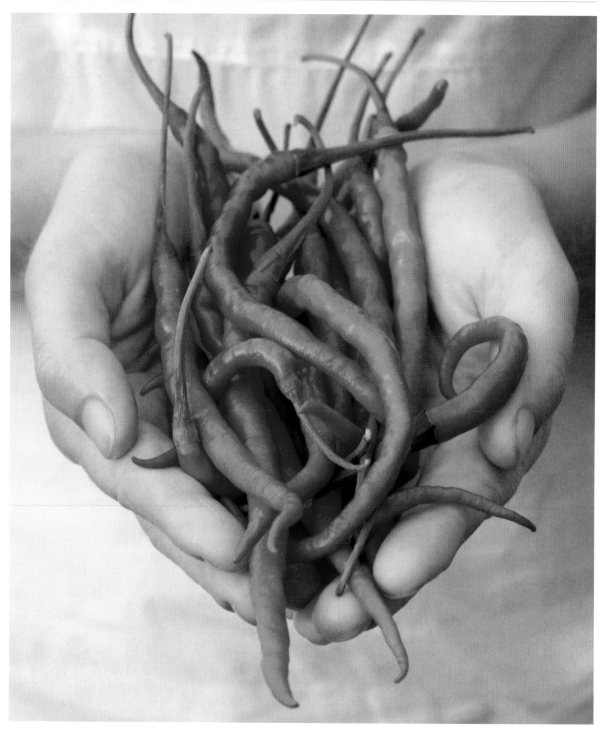

So how can we fight back?

Some foods can minimise the likelihood of inflammation and help the weight-controlling hormones to do what they do best: control our appetite and balance our blood sugar. These include fruits, vegetables, oily fish, nuts and seeds and their oils, wholegrains and herbs and spices.

Herbal helpers

Herbs and spices are important because they are rich in antioxidants, substances that protect body cells from the damage created when the inflammatory process is in full swing. Antioxidants are like protective parents that form a shield around our body's cells and absorb free radicals, which lose their destructive energy and are safely excreted from the body.

If you cut an apple in half and leave one half uncovered for 20 minutes you can see free radical damage occurring. The apple starts to go brown and dries up because it reacts with the oxygen in the air causing free radicals to be formed. If you soak the other half in lemon juice however, it retains its white colour and texture. This is because it has been protected by the vitamin C in lemon juice. Vitamin C is a powerful antioxidant.

The antioxidant-rich, anti-inflammatory properties of herbs and spices encourage fat burning while reducing fat storage. They also add flavour and excitement to food, which results in reduced salt consumption. Too much salt prompts fluid retention, another fat-loss adversary.

Herbs and spices included in the 2-week diet:

- Black pepper
- Cayenne
- Chilli
- Cinnamon
- Cumin
- Garlic
- Ginger
- Mint
- Mustard
- Oregano
- Parsley
- Rosemary
- Thyme
- Turmeric

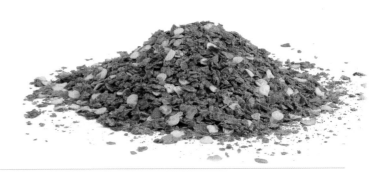

Pink seafood

When it comes to choosing your seafood, think pink to burn fat

Ever wondered what gives salmon, prawns, langoustine, lobster and their pink swimming companions their colour? No, us neither – but we should. It's down to a carotenoid called astaxanthin; and research suggests that this naturally occurring chemical may be the most powerful antioxidant yet to go under the microscope.

It has been shown to provide the body with an internal sunscreen, protecting us from the damaging effects of UV rays. This exciting discovery has already led to astaxanthin being included in anti-ageing skincare and sunscreens.

Astaxanthin has also been shown to increase the usage of fat as an energy source and accelerate fat-burning during exercise. Japanese researchers recently demonstrated that mice given astaxanthin along with a high-fat diet had significantly lower body weight and body fat levels compared to mice fed on a high-fat diet alone.

In another study, mice were given astaxanthin along with a daily exercise routine. After four weeks, they showed increased fat usage during exercise. At present, no human studies have been concluded, but researchers are confident that this powerful pink substance may play an important role in the fight against our expanding waistlines.

It's good for the gut, too!

There is another reason why astaxanthin is a valuable addition to a diet focused on fat loss: its role in good gastric health. Inflammation of the gut is on the increase and a condition known as leaky gut syndrome is largely to blame.

The digestive tract consists of a long tube, which connects the mouth to the anus. After food is swallowed it passes through the oesophagus to the stomach, where enzymes break it down into tiny particles. These then pass into the small intestine, the major function of which is to absorb the valuable nutrients and release them into the bloodstream. Next, the food particles are passed to the liver for further processing to produce the essentials, which are quickly delivered to cells to provide the energy to make new cells, repair cells and generally keep us in good health.

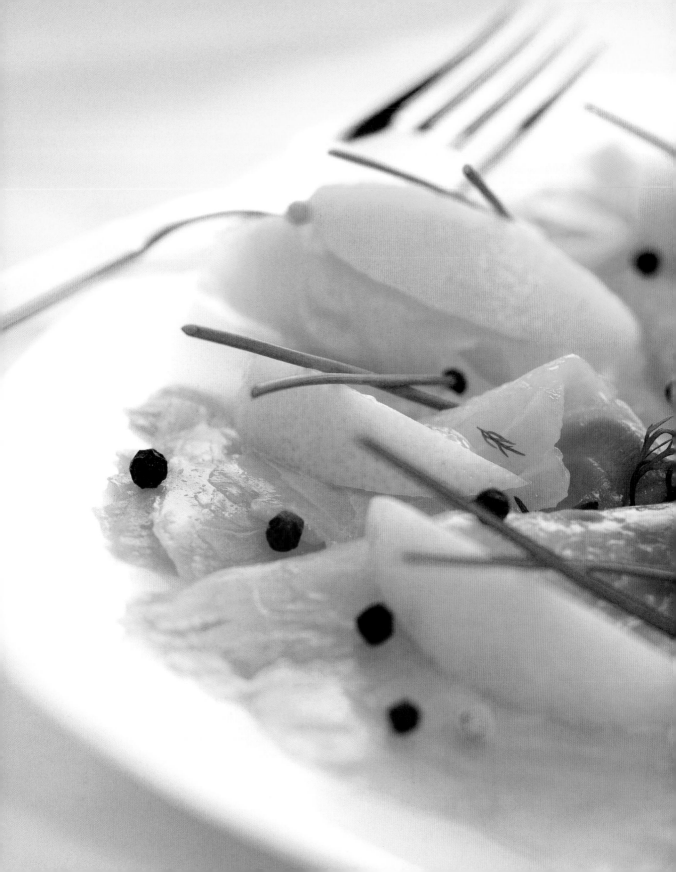

The inner lining of the small intestine can, however, become inflamed due to infection, toxic substances within foods, or as a result of the over-consumption of processed fats, sugars and food additives. Over time, this weakens the small intestine's permeability and the gut becomes leaky. This allows overly large, damaging food molecules to enter the bloodstream; causing an immediate response by the immune system, which recognises these invaders as a threat to health.

As they pass through the liver they have to be detoxified to limit the potential damage, but this puts stress on its detoxification capability. As a result, the toxins are being only partially processed and allowed to build up. In a bid to restore its health and efficiency and prevent these partially-processed toxins from being released into the bloodstream, the liver is forced to pack them up and send them off for safe storage – and our fat cells are only too willing to accommodate!

It is hard enough to encourage fat cells to release their energy and shrink, but it is even harder when they are storing toxins which, when released into the bloodstream, are likely to create havoc and compromise our health. This is the body's damage limitation at its best, but can be a major stumbling block when we want to shift fat.

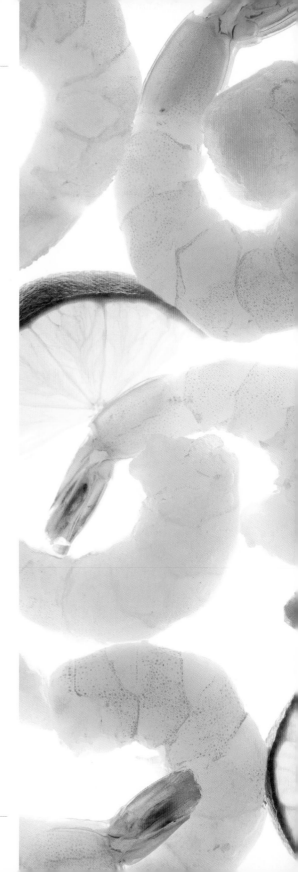

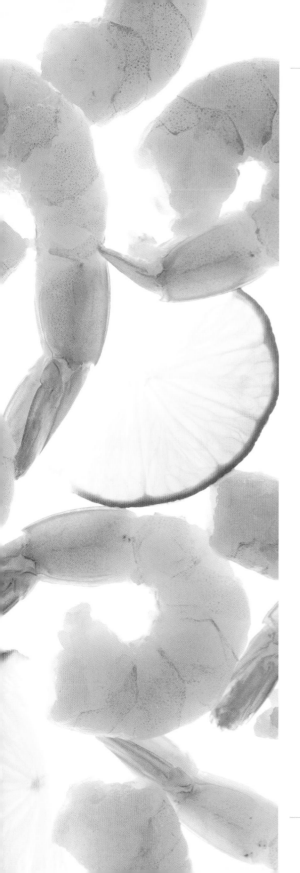

Fat loss becomes a whole lot easier, quicker and more maintainable when the cells that line the small intestine are healthy and strong. Astaxanthin has not only shown itself to be protective of the outer membranes of these cells, reducing the chance of toxic substances compromising their permeability, but also has the ability to mount a massive anti-inflammatory effect should toxic substances sneak through into the bloodstream. This is clearly a substance that is earning its stripes as a fat-loss warrior.

Pink seafood included in the 2-week diet:
- Crab
- Crayfish
- Lobster
- Prawns
- Rainbow trout
- Red caviar
- Salmon
- Shrimps

Dopamine

It doesn't *burn fat* per se, but dopamine is the key to curbing those cravings

Depriving ourselves of foods that give us pleasure is perhaps one of the most documented reasons dieters give up after relatively short periods. If we don't feed our desires, we wither. The key to getting pleasure is dopamine, a neurotransmitter that helps control the brain's reward and happiness centre. The chemical messages it communicates to the brain regulate emotional responses that lead us to not only seek reward, but also to take action to move towards it.

Several studies indicate that people who are overweight produce low levels of dopamine, so they're unconsciously driven to seek ways to raise the level with food to get the feel-good factor back. The quickest way to restore levels is by eating foods that release their sugars rapidly, but these foods invariably lead to further weight gain. Worse still, repeated consumption desensitises the receptors in the brain, which means more of the same is required to get the reward we seek.

Dose up on dopamine

To stop us reaching for the Häagen-Dazs, we have to find ways to increase dopamine levels naturally. One is through exercise. Among the early changes seen when people start an aerobic training programme are mood elevation, heightened energy levels, enhanced self-confidence and self-esteem, lower anxiety levels, resistance to depression and improved coping ability.

Higher levels of dopamine have been recorded following aerobic exercise training in several studies, and there is also evidence that levels remain elevated for longer. It has yet to be ascertained whether certain types of aerobic exercise achieve higher levels than others, or indeed whether levels stay elevated for longer dependent on the time of day we exercise. But one thing is for sure: findings so far present another good reason to get physical on a daily basis.

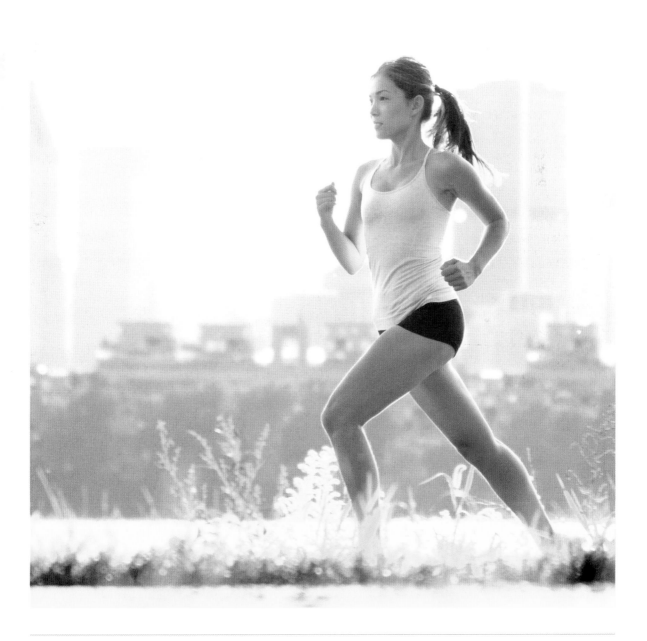

Feel-good foods

The brain cells that manufacture dopamine use phenylalanine as the raw material. Phenylalanine is an essential amino acid found in the brain and blood plasma, which can convert in the body to tyrosine, another amino acid that in turn is used to synthesise dopamine. Amino acids are the building blocks of protein, so to encourage good levels of dopamine, we need to eat protein foods, particularly those rich in phenylalanine and tyrosine.

We also need good levels of certain vitamins and minerals, which feed the enzymes (catalysts) that promote the production of dopamine. Iron, copper, folic acid and vitamins B3, B6 and C are the important ones, and they're all supplied in good amounts in *The Ultimate 2-Week Fat Loss Diet*.

Feel-good foods included in the 2-week diet:
- Bananas
- Chicken
- Chickpeas
- Eggs
- Fish
- Lentils
- Oats
- Peanuts
- Pumpkin seeds
- Sesame seeds
- Shellfish
- Turkey
- Venison

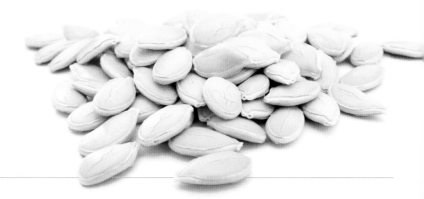

Fat-loss boosters

Did you know?
Sex is not only a great stress-reliever, but it burns around 6-7kcals per minute. Fat burning, physically demanding *and* fun... what's not to love?

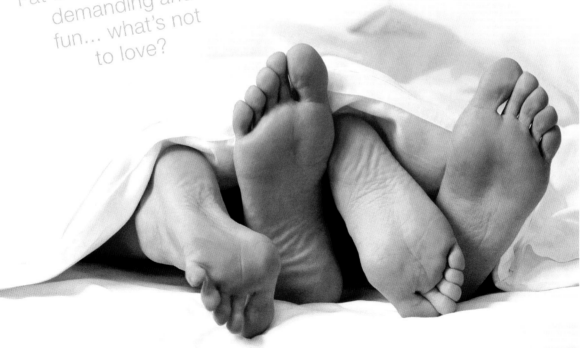

Alcohol and caffeine

Here's how to turn traditional diet enemies into fat-loss friends

Alcohol

We've all beaten ourselves up for having that extra glass of cab sav at some stage. But the good news is, it might not have been as bad for us as we think. Evidence suggests that drinking two to four glasses of red wine a day reduces the risk of a heart attack by up to 32 per cent, due to the protective combination of the alcohol and the antioxidant resveratrol. Music to the ears of those of us partial to the occasional glass or two; but can the odd drink also feature in a fat-loss diet?

If you don't currently drink alcohol, don't take it up in a bid to cut your risk of heart disease; a healthy diet and lifestyle will take care of that. Or, if you are a heavy drinker, you should try to cut back to avoid serious health problems. But, in some cases, alcohol can indeed be part of a weight-loss plan. It has a lot to do with what we drink, when we drink, how much we drink and what we eat before, during and after our favourite tipple.

Moderation is the key

People who drink moderately (max two units per day for men, one unit for women), are able to spread their consumption through the week and don't have any of the absolute reasons why we shouldn't be drinking alcohol (pregnancy, on medication, operating heavy machinery, poor health history etc) can take comfort in the fact that enjoying some downtime with glass in hand may well have a few benefits.

Studies have found that adults with moderate alcohol intakes have around a 30 per cent lower risk of developing type 2 diabetes than teetotallers. It has been suggested this may be associated with improved insulin sensitivity. But what is insulin sensitivity and why is it so important for fat loss?

Insulin sensitivity

The hormone insulin is produced by the pancreas and monitors the level of glucose (sugar) in the bloodstream by continually transporting it to our body cells to create energy. But, when this sugar-monitoring mechanism has to deal with a repeated flood of glucose from foods that require very little processing (sugary cereals, cakes, biscuits, pastries, alcohol, fizzy drinks and the rest), it becomes stressed, considers throwing in the towel and demands time out.

The pancreas becomes overworked, the body cells become less receptive and the whole system becomes less efficient. The possible results? Scenario 1 is that the pancreas produces less and less insulin, and type 2 diabetes develops. Scenario 2 is that the cells take in less

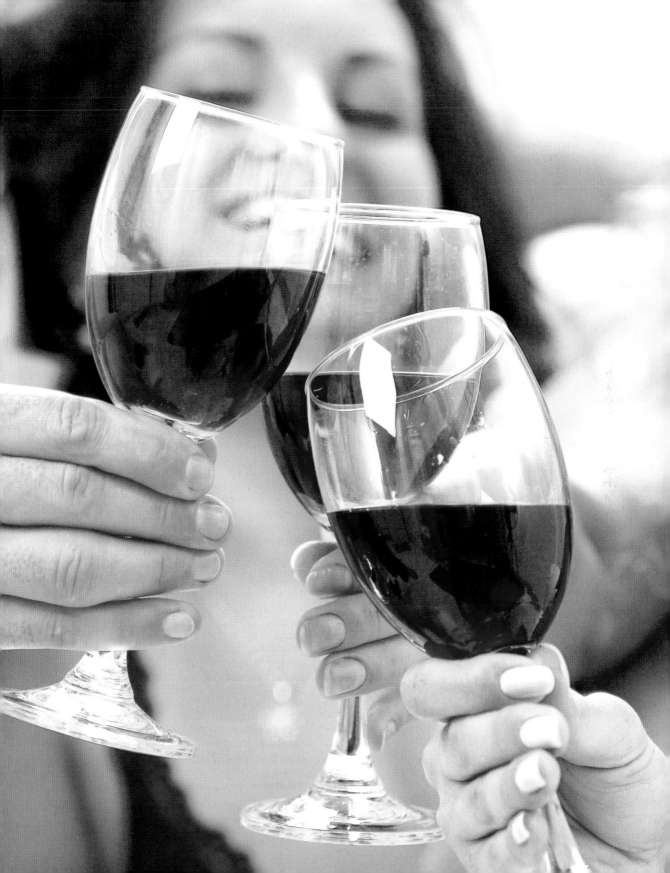

and less glucose, causing abnormally high levels of insulin in the blood (hyperinsulinemia), which can lead to high blood pressure, high levels of damaging cholesterol and heart disease. Either one is to be avoided, due to the well documented, debilitating health issues.

How to reap the benefits of alcohol

So, we want to enjoy the insulin-sensitising benefits of alcohol, but skip the weight-gain risk. How? The best advice is to have a glass of good red wine with your evening meal (cabernet sauvignon, pinot noir and merlot are richest in protective flavonoids) and only occasionally have another.

But if your social life is full of meals out and entertaining at home, try these tricks to minimise the calories without meaning you have to say 'no' to invitations:

Always have a protein-rich snack before or with a drink. Alcohol raises blood sugar very quickly, so snack on a couple of oatcakes with nut butter, a small pot of live natural yoghurt with fresh fruit, a chicken leg, a cold boiled egg, some crunchy baby vegetables with a small pot of houmous or a handful of almonds to help moderate the sugar spike.

— For every drink you have, have two large glasses of water. This will seriously cut the amount of alcohol you drink. Alcohol dehydrates, so have a few glasses of water before bed (and keep another one by the bed) to help the body to rehydrate and ensure you feel fresh the next morning.

Alcohol increases your appetite, lessens your resolve and removes your inhibitions, so always make sure you have a friend/partner around to keep you on track.

— Avoid fizzy mixers at all costs – they are full of sugar. The 'diet' alternatives are no better, they just increase your desire for more sugar and consequently more alcohol.

— Avoid all lite beers, alcopops and ready-mixed spirit-based cocktails – sugar, sugar and yet more sugar!

— Aim for good quality wine, or clear spirits like vodka, gin or white rum served on the rocks or with natural, unsweetened fruit juices.

— Cocktails can be dangerous and are often high in sugar, but if you stick to Breezes, Martinis, Sours, Manhattans, Screwdrivers, Punches and Pimms (no sugar added, just the sweetness from the fruit), you shouldn't get into too much trouble. And, don't forget the highly nutritious, satisfying and delicious Bloody Mary or Bloody Caesar.

— Mix white wine with soda water to make it last twice as long and halve the calories. If you can't bear to dilute it, opt for dry whites as these contain fewer calories than their sweeter counterparts.

— Follow in the footsteps of celebrities and enjoy a glass of bubbly if funds allow. In general you drink less as it's served in smaller glasses and the bubbles fill you up.

— Most measures of spirits poured at home are larger than those served in bars and pubs, with the result that your drink will probably contain twice as many calories. If you do a lot of entertaining at home, it's worth investing in a spirits measure. Also, always pour spirits into the glass before adding ice or mixers, so you can actually see just how much alcohol is involved.

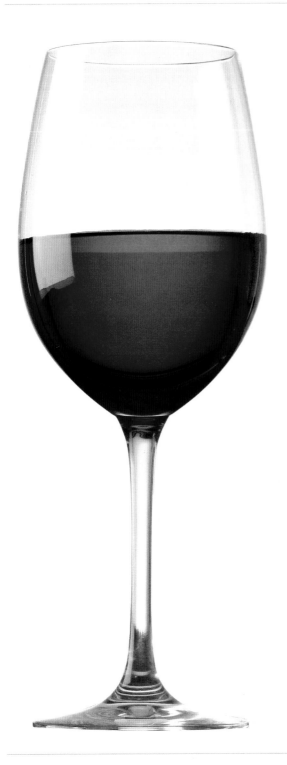

Steer clear of beer, lager and cider as they're loaded with calories. And the higher the alcohol content, the more calories drinks contain. For example, a pint of standard beer contains around 160 calories, whereas a bottle of strong lager can contain more like 220 calories.

Beware of trendy wine bars. Many serve spirits in double measures as the standard, with the result that you get double the calories. Some pubs also serve 35ml measures of spirits rather than 25ml measures and so also contain more calories. Finally, watch out for huge wine glasses – some are so large that a glass of wine may actually be closer to a third of a bottle.

Avoid creamy liqueurs after dinner and instead have a single shot of brandy if you really fancy ending your meal with a drink. Most cream-based liqueurs contain around 80-100 calories per 25ml measure compared with 50 calories in a single brandy.

Remember that happy hours are designed to get you to drink more and keep you in the same place all night. Unfortunately, this means while the bar gains pounds, so do you as you indulge in far more drinks than you would during other hours.

Why not offer to drive from time to time? Your partner will really appreciate it, and you won't be able to drink anything other than fresh fruit and vegetable juices, sparkling water or soda and lime!

CAFFEINE

t's hard to find a coffee lover who can bin the cappuccino habit long term, but there is evidence to suggest it may not be the fat-loss foe it was believed to be. Bodybuilders and athletes have been using caffeine to reduce body fat for more than 20 years, but it is only recently that its fat-burning properties have been further investigated. As with alcohol, it's all about the what, the when and the how.

Properly used, caffeine stimulates the central nervous system, increases the use of body fat as fuel and preserves glycogen levels (the glucose stored in the liver and muscles). But it is also a diuretic, so it promotes the loss of water from our body cells and raises body temperature, so we overheat.

Studies on professional athletes reveal that caffeine taken three hours before exercise allowed them to perform longer and harder before exhaustion. It also increased the use of fat for fuel, sparing the glycogen energy supplies in the muscles, which, when depleted, causes the exhaustion commonly known as 'hitting the wall'. But, few of us are professional athletes, so how can caffeine play a role in fat burning for us, too?

The upsides

Caffeine increases the number of calories the body burns at rest. A single 100mg dose of caffeine can increase our metabolic rate by three to four per cent for at least an hour and a half afterwards. Consuming 100mg every two hours for 12 hours has also been shown to increase our daily metabolic rate by up to 11 per cent (one cup of reasonably strong coffee contains anywhere between 65 and 115mg of caffeine). However, it doesn't have the same effect in everyone. The rise in the metabolic rate is around 150 calories in lean individuals, but only around 80 calories for those who are overweight.

One study compared the effects of caffeine in 10 lean and 10 obese women. The rise in metabolic rate following the consumption of caffeine was just under five per cent in the obese women and just over seven per cent in the lean women. Although the effect on their metabolic rate could no longer be seen the following day, both groups were still burning between 10 per cent and 30 per cent more fat at rest than before the caffeine trial.

The downsides

Before you start lining up the lattes, it's important to note that we're not suggesting you drink a cup of coffee every two hours over a 12-hour period! Coffee has quite a few downsides:

— Many of the chemicals in coffee irritate the stomach lining, causing an increase of stomach acid, which can lead to digestive disorders
— It raises blood pressure
— It decreases quality of sleep
— It causes problems with blood sugar control
— It stimulates the intestines, resulting in shortened transit times for food and less absorption of nutrients
— It stimulates more frequent urination and subsequent loss of various vitamins and minerals
— It leaches calcium from the bones increasing the risk of osteoporosis
— It is one of most heavily pesticide-sprayed crops

However, caffeine does have a role to play in fat loss. When used in conjunction with a healthy lifestyle, it can make losing fat a little faster and a little easier, particularly when consumed before exercise.

How to give fat a caffeine kick

Have a double espresso or a small cup of strong filtered coffee first thing in the morning, then get out for a brisk walk, jog or run for 30 minutes. Have at least one large glass of water when you get back home, shower and dress then have a breakfast with plenty of fruit.

Try substituting your mid-morning coffee with a cup of green tea, a rich source of caffeine that doesn't pose the health risks of coffee and doesn't involve milk or sugar. And, whatever you do, don't resort to caffeinated fizzy drinks in a bid to boost your caffeine levels and increase fat burning; there are around eight spoonfuls of sugar in every can!

Brown fat cells

Not all fats are bad! Know friend from foe to give your metabolism a boost

Most body fat is white fat, the bulky stuff that stores excess calories, makes up cell membranes, insulates nerve cells, cushions our organs and sits on our hips. But we also have small amounts of brown fat. These fat cells not only have a much richer blood supply, but are packed with mitochondria, the body's energy powerhouses.

This makes them a great deal more metabolically active, and instead of making energy, they make *heat*, using white fat and glucose from the bloodstream for fuel. This means that basal metabolic rate (BMR) increases and more calories are burned. Some studies estimate that active brown cells can burn up as much as 20 per cent of our daily calorie intake.

How can we boost brown fat?

We are born with a good supply, and as babies we have the ability to turn white fat cells into brown fat cells to keep the body warm. Sadly, as we age the process becomes less efficient; and it was thought that we lose all of it as we age. However, new research has discovered that adults *do* retain some brown fat, and that brown fat is inversely proportional to body mass index (BMI). Researchers now think that increasing our brown fat activity may help us lose weight.

There are ways you can help to enhance brown fat activity. Keeping cool is one of them: sitting in a chilly room, wearing fewer clothes, turning the thermostat down and running the shower on cool for a minute can all activate brown fat, but the researchers cautioned that it is not yet clear whether that would translate to weight loss.

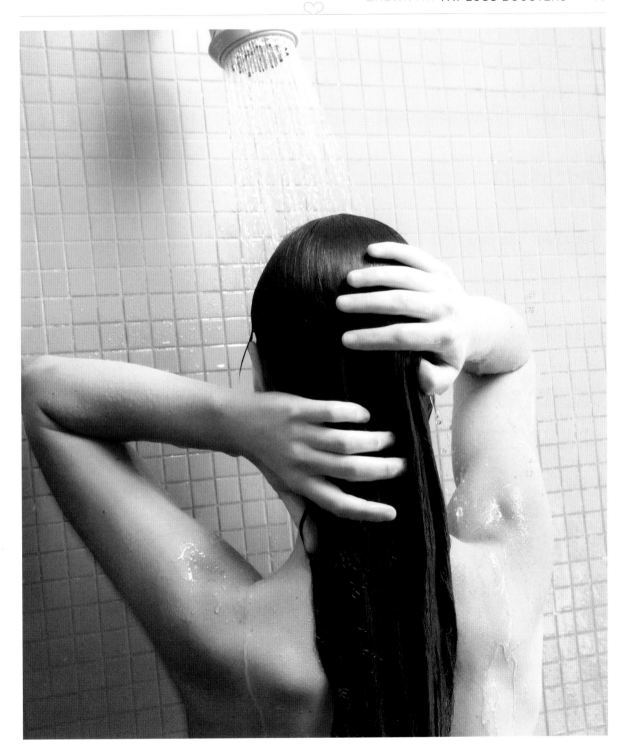

Sex, sleep and sunshine

Let's hear it for these fun ways to lose fat…

Sex

Anti-ageing researchers have proposed that people showing the slowest ageing rates often have a particularly well-developed libido and sex life. The main libido-determining hormone is testosterone, and, while women don't want this sex hormone to dominate, men don't want it to underachieve, so healthy levels are the goal for both sexes. An added bonus is that this hormone is a fat-burner when certain vitamins and minerals are supplied through our diet, so it's not just about eating more oysters!

Why testosterone burns fat

Like a car, fat cells have brakes and accelerators. The parts of a fat cell that accelerate the release of fat are called beta receptors, while the parts of a fat cell that put the brakes on fat loss are known as alpha receptors. Beta receptors help fat loss because they increase the rate at which stored fat is broken down as well as increasing blood flow in fat tissue. In contrast, alpha receptors hinder fat loss, slowing the flow of fat out of the cells. The distribution of these brakes and accelerators explains, to a degree, why we lose body fat faster in certain parts of the body than in others.

If a fat cell has more beta receptors, it releases stored fat more quickly, and this is where testosterone appears to help. It can increase the number of beta receptors, making it easier to lose stored fat. It has also been shown to limit fat storage; when fat cells are exposed to testosterone in a test tube, the activity of the enzyme that promotes fat storage, synthase, is dramatically reduced.

Foods that balance testosterone levels in the 2-week diet:
— Apples
— Broccoli
— Chickpeas
— Eggs
— Garlic and onions
— Green leafy vegetables
— Lean beef
— Olives
— Peanuts
— Red peppers

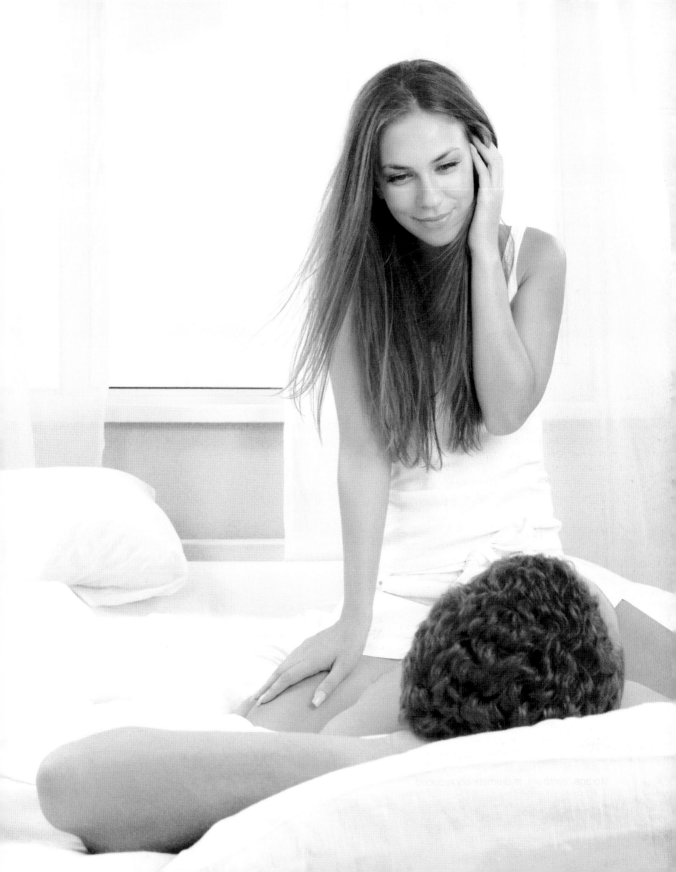

Sleep

A number of studies have found that those who get less than six hours of sleep per night tend to gain more weight over time than people who get seven to eight hours. The production of two hormones, leptin and grehlin, which control hunger and fullness, are influenced by how much or how little sleep we get.

Leptin is produced by the fat cells and controls appetite by telling the brain when energy stores are replenished and we've had enough to eat. Grehlin is produced in the stomach and controls hunger, by telling the brain when we are hungry and need nourishment. When these hormones are working optimally we are better able to control when we eat and how much we eat; but unfortunately they are easily disrupted. If the signals to the brain are scrambled, it's all too easy to just go along with our desires, meaning we gorge rather than graze, and pile on the pounds.

Snooze to lose fat

Leptin levels peak when we are asleep, so if we don't get enough sleep, levels drop. If we are regularly sleep deprived, leptin stays low and the brain interprets this as a reduction in energy stores, prompting us to eat more in an effort to get the balance back. Continued lack of sleep also causes grehlin levels to rise, which means our appetite is repeatedly stimulated and we want more food. The two combined set the stage for overeating, so getting our eight hours a night is critical.

Sleep easier

But what if you are one of the millions for whom a good night's sleep is the goal but rarely a reality? You either can't get to sleep and toss and turn for hours, or you wake up in the early hours and can't get back to sleep; your leptin and grehlin levels are all over the place and fat loss isn't going to be easy. So what can you do?

Have a bedtime snack that includes foods that encourage the production of the sleep-inducing neurotransmitter, serotonin. When you are trying to shift fat, the suggestion that you should eat before you hit the sack may sound strange, but when you understand that sleep deprivation promotes weight gain, it is well worth reconsidering.

Our serotonin levels are directly related to the amount of tryptophan (an essential amino acid found in protein foods) in the blood: as our levels of tryptophan in the brain rise and fall, so do our levels of serotonin. Tryptophan can be the runt of the litter when it comes to competing with the other amino acids to get from the bloodstream into the brain, but a little carbohydrate added to a protein-rich snack creates a diversion, allowing tryptophan to take the stage.

Foods that boost serotonin in the 2-week diet:
— Bananas
— Cottage cheese
— Dark chocolate
— Lemon juice
— Lettuce
— Oats
— Peanuts
— Rye
— Soya milk
— Turkey
— Yoghurt

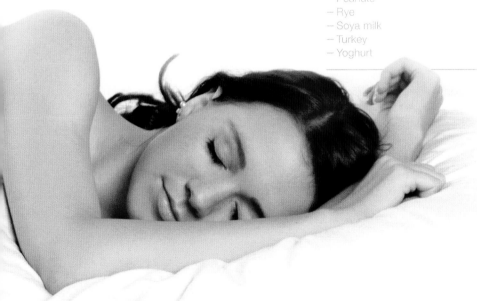

Sunshine

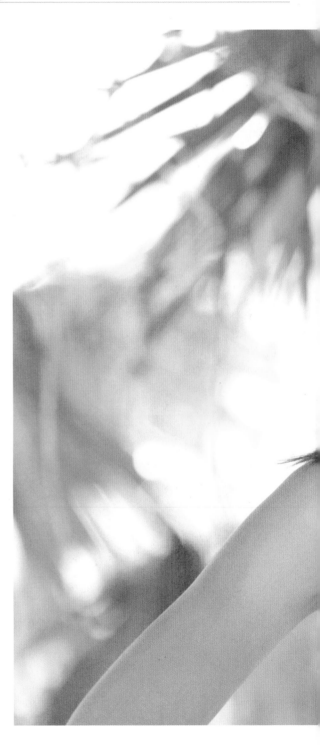

Vitamin D, which is essential for the absorption of calcium into our bones to keep them strong, is produced within the body when we are exposed to sunlight. However, recent research reveals that many of us are deficient in this vitamin, and that women who are D-deficient carry between 40 per cent and 80 per cent more abdominal fat than their D-rich counterparts. Now is definitely the time to become D-aware!

D is for destroying fat

As previously discussed, fat cells are not just storage depots; they are metabolically active. Vitamin D, which is stored in fat cells, has an important role in regulating how much fat we store and how much we burn. We know that leptin, the hormone that controls appetite, is produced by the fat cells and tells the brain when we have had enough to eat; but it appears that vitamin D deficiency can interfere with this appetite-suppressing hormone.

Because vitamin D is stored in fat cells, one would imagine that the bigger our fat cells, the more vitamin D we are able to store, allowing its release into the bloodstream for bone building and cellular health. But quite the opposite has been noted. The fatter we are, the higher our risk of D-deficiency because vitamin D gets locked inside fat cells and becomes unavailable for use.

In one study, a group of obese adults (with BMIs above 30) and a group of lean adults (with BMIs of 19-24) were exposed to the same amount of UVB rays. Blood levels of vitamin D in the lean adults rose by almost double those in their obese counterparts. This indicates that when we are overweight we need a lot more D.

Vitamin D deficiency has also been shown to disrupt the delicate balance of insulin production by the pancreas and increase the possibility of insulin resistance. Over time, this can lead not only to weight gain but also to an increased risk of type 2 diabetes.

How to dose up on D

Vitamin D is primarily synthesised in the skin after exposure to sunshine. As little as five to 10 minutes of sun exposure on arms, legs and face three times a week without

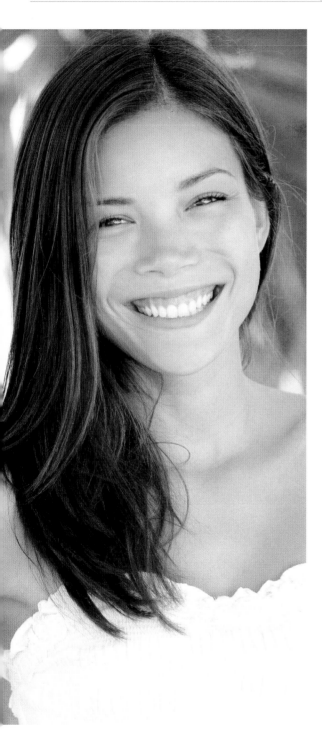

sunscreen, between 11am and 2pm during the spring, summer, and autumn, should provide a light-skinned individual with adequate vitamin D. Those with dark skin are thought to require twice or three times the exposure.

However, a recent UK survey indicates that more than half of the adult population is deficient in vitamin D and, in the winter, about one in six people show a severe deficiency. If the body cannot produce enough vitamin D because of insufficient sunlight exposure, we need to up our levels with D-rich foods.

How much do we need?

A new report has found that a minimum of 4,000IU of vitamin D is required daily to maintain optimal blood levels. Around 3,500 men and women had their vitamin D levels measured and completed online surveys to monitor vitamin D status and health outcomes over five years. The aim of this study was to assess how much vitamin D is needed to ensure optimal rather than just adequate levels in the average person.

The researchers found that daily intakes of between 4,000IU and 8,000IU are needed to maintain blood levels of vitamin D and reduce the risk of diseases such as breast cancer, colon cancer, multiple sclerosis and type 1 diabetes. They also found this dose was very safe.

So, daily exposure to sunlight and a diet packed with foods rich in vitamin D is crucial. You may also wish to have your D levels checked; a simple blood test is available from your GP. If the sunshine and the D-rich foods don't see you reaching the mark, supplementation may be required.

Vitamin D-rich foods in the 2-week diet:
– Eggs
– Herring
– Mackerel
– Sardines
– Tinned salmon

CHANGE

YOUR REFLECTION

Diet Protein is arguably the most sophisticated diet protein shake available today. Reflex Nutrition have used the latest advances in protein and weight loss technology to bring you a product that's specifically designed to help you achieve a healthy, well defined and toned body.

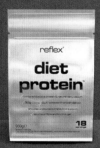

RRP £32.99
900g - 18 x 50g servings

One serving of Reflex Diet Protein provides 3.2 grams of Clarinol™ CLA, a research based dose proven to help reduce body fat primarily in the abdomen and particularly in women, the legs.

Each serving of Reflex Diet Protein is packed with additional diet support. Green Tea extract is added for its long standing reputation for aiding dieters.

Diet Protein contains no added sugar or maltodextrin. It's perfect for dieters wanting to restrict their carbohydrate content.

Diet Protein comes in a variety of mouthwatering flavours. All of which have been up against a taste test panel to ensure that they are the best tasting diet shakes on the market.

Find out more about our products at:

www.reflex-nutrition.com

 Please visit & join our Facebook page at Reflex Nutrition Ltd

 @ReflexNutrition

ecotricity

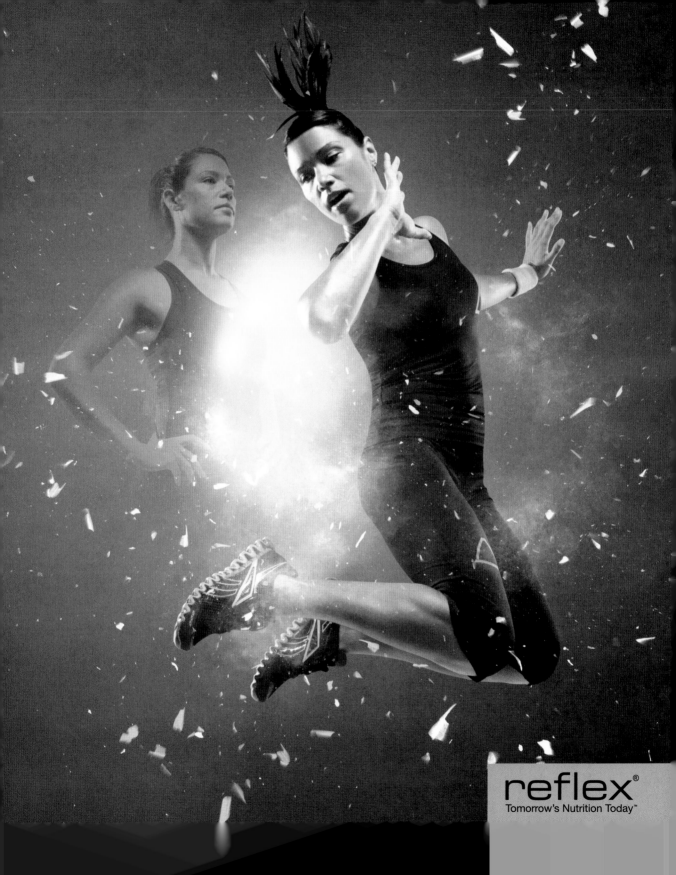

reflex®
Tomorrow's Nutrition Today™

Exercise

Yes, your diet is important, but if you *really* want to blast the fat, it's time to get fit

Sure, the main aim of this book is to understand how we can whittle our waistlines with the foods we eat. But it's also important to get up to date with the latest ways to blast fat with exercise. Let's face it, most of us don't want to spend hours in the gym doing the same old routine, we're probably short of time, and total dedication is tough. So here are the best ways to shift fat, fast.

Resistance training

What is it?

Strength-building exercises using dumbbells, exercise machines, your own body weight, bottles of water, or an elastic band as resistance. Examples include biceps curls, leg presses and press-ups.

What does it do?

Resistance training accelerates fat burning because there is an increased secretion of growth hormone (GH) and noradrenaline, two hormones that help mobilise fat stores and use fat for fuel. More calories are expended during the intense workout and your BMR (basal metabolic rate) is increased for many hours after you have finished training, which is when the fat burning kicks in.

How do I do it?

When you exercise using any kind of weights, muscles are strengthened by pitting each group against a force (resistance). To develop a muscle you must work all the fibres within it, which means pushing them to their limit for short periods of time, resting them briefly, then repeating the process. You should work with a weight heavy enough to make the last few repetitions difficult to perform.

This is not the kind of exercise where you chat to a friend while you work out. It requires concentration and determination. When a muscle is overloaded, lactic acid is produced causing the burn in the muscle that ultimately leads to muscular fatigue – you have to push past that sensation and ensure your mind doesn't give up before your body. The rest between repetitions enables the lactic acid to be flushed from the bloodstream, allowing the muscles to be refreshed before working them again.

Recommendations vary, but generally 30-40 minutes of resistance exercise three times a week is a good goal. To allow the muscles to repair and regenerate, 48 hours should be allowed between sessions. This allows protein synthesis (the process by which the body repairs muscle tissue) to take place, preventing injury.

What if I've never done it before?

It's never too late to start. In a study of elderly men and women (average age 87) who lifted weights three times a week for 10 weeks, muscle strength increased by a 113 per cent on average. This improvement in strength let them walk 12 per cent faster than before, climb 28 per cent more stairs and lose excess body fat. So it really is *never* too late.

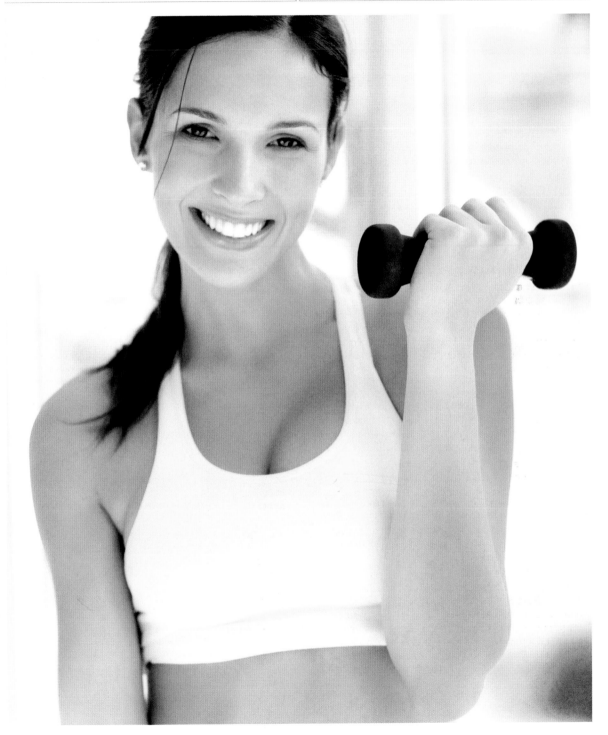

Interval training

What is it?

A way of doing aerobic exercise that alternates one minute of intense effort with one to four minutes of lower-intensity work. An example would be alternating sprints with steady jogging.

What does it do?

Aerobic exercise helps the cardiovascular system become more efficient at delivering oxygen to working muscles, delaying the lactic acid build-up and letting you train at a higher level of intensity. Aerobic exercise also expands the network of blood vessels that allows nutrients to be absorbed into body tissues, so muscles can repair more effectively. This expanded network of blood vessels also helps to clear waste products, particularly carbon dioxide from the food-burning process. Efficient exchange of oxygen and nutrients for carbon dioxide and waste equals a fit and healthy body.

What's more, the mitochondria (the body's energy factories) expand in size and number and require more energy. Once they have used up the glycogen (the stored glucose within the muscle cells and the liver), they call on the fat cells to release energy – meaning you burn off the bulge.

Why interval training?

Interval training provides significant benefits over steady state exercise (e.g. a steady 30-minute jog) and is more effective at burning fat because the fat-burning is prolonged after activity. During the intense phase, the lactic acid builds up quickly and during the less intense phase it is cleared from the blood and oxygen stores are replenished.

How do I do it?

If you are a jogger, run as fast and as hard as you can for one minute then reduce your speed to a steady jog for between one and four minutes. Keep repeating until 30 minutes is up. You can use this pattern for any kind of aerobic exercise, such as rowing, cycling, swimming, skipping or using a mini trampoline – just go as hard as you can cope with for one minute, then bring it down to a manageable pace for four minutes. A mere five repetitions later and your 30 minutes of cardio are done! As you get fitter you can reduce the number of minutes between the intense phases during the middle section of your workout.

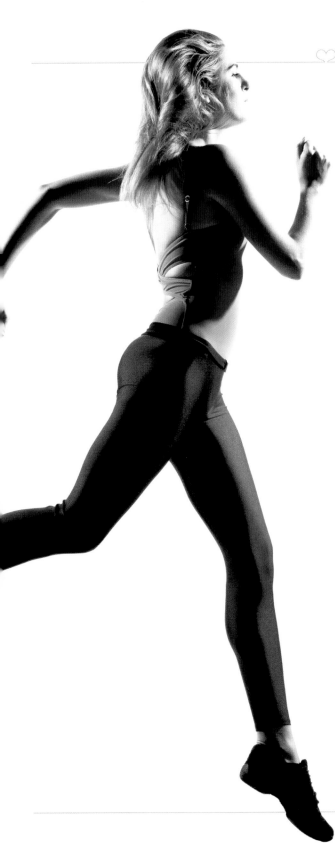

When intervals meet resistance...

Resistance training for 30 minutes on Monday, Wednesday and Friday (or Tuesday, Thursday and Saturday) and interval training for 30 minutes on the other three days, with one day of rest, suits many peoples' timetables. You may prefer to do both in a one-hour workout only three times a week (with one rest day between each).

So which should you do first? Resistance followed by intervals appears to have the edge. Since the body's preferred energy source is glucose, that's what we should target first – and resistance training does that.

Resistance training is an anaerobic exercise, where the body gets its fuel first from the glucose from carbohydrates in the bloodstream, then from stored glucose in the muscles and liver. It uses minimal oxygen, and as fat can only be burned in the presence of oxygen, the fat cells won't be mobilised into releasing their energy stores until we stop.

By the time we embark on the interval training, glycogen stores are pretty well used up and, because it is aerobic (i.e. uses lots of oxygen) the body will have to call on the fat stores for energy. Plus, the high intensity of both sessions means the body will continue to burn calories for many hours afterwards.

Unfit or unused to exercise?

Don't worry, the principles of resistance and interval training apply no matter where you start. Resistance training is all about introducing some weights into your life; and if you want to start with a couple of cans of baked beans you will still be creating the force.

Similarly, interval training is all about moving as fast as you can manage for one minute followed by four minutes of slowing the pace. Walking is a great way to start – brisk for one minute, less intense for four. As you get fitter, your body will get acclimatised and you can push the intensity.

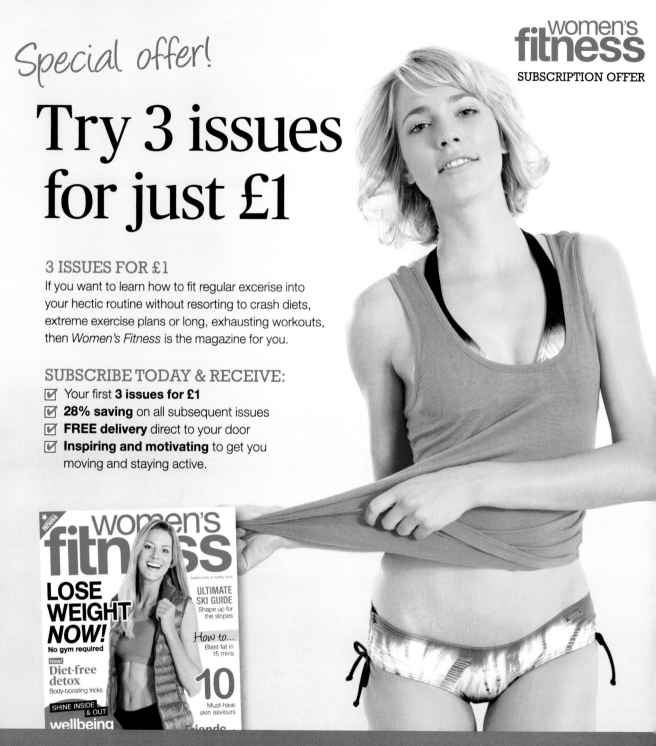

Sneaky secrets for success

Fire up your fat loss with these tried-and-tested tricks

So, we've looked at nutrition and exercise, but for an extra cherry on the weight-loss cake, try some of these tried-and-tested strategies from successful dieters. Some make biochemical sense, some are brilliant coping techniques and others are just plain wacky – but they work!

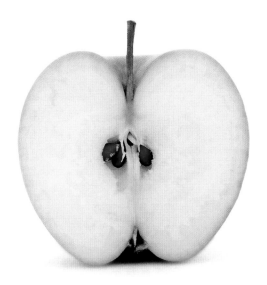

 I always have three apples and a bag of almonds in my handbag

Why it works: Apples (and pears) are high in pectin, which helps reduce fat absorption; and they're rich in soluble fibre, which slows down the absorption of sugars into the bloodstream. Almonds are a great protein/essential fat combination. The two together make for a balanced, fat-burning and filling snack; perfect on the go.

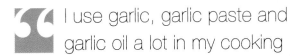 I use garlic, garlic paste and garlic oil a lot in my cooking

Why it works: Garlic contains a substance called allicin, which research has shown to have a significant protective effect on cells, helping to reduce fatty deposits. Garlic and onions (also rich in allicin) have been linked to increasing our metabolic rate and insulin sensitivity. You can experiment with garlic capsules to reduce any odour-related issues!

'I can't give up cheese, so I only eat it at the weekend'
Why it works: Full-fat cheeses are high in calories and saturated fat, so they can pile on the pounds. Having them as a weekend treat means you don't deprive yourself of something you love but you stay on track.

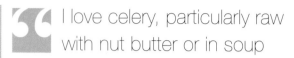
I love celery, particularly raw with nut butter or in soup

Why it works: Celery is very low in calories and, because it is also high in fibre, the body burns more calories than it uses to digest it; this is known as diet-induced thermogenesis, or DIT. Vegetables with less fibre and more water such as lettuce, peeled or canned vegetables and vegetable juices don't require the same amount of energy.

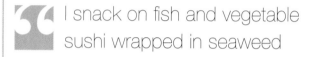
I snack on fish and vegetable sushi wrapped in seaweed

Why it works: Seaweed is rich in iodine, which feeds the thyroid gland, a major player in maintaining an efficient metabolism. You might also wish to try kelp salt granules as an alternative to regular salt. They are rich in iodine, low in sodium and high in potassium, magnesium and other mineral salts, which reduce the risk of high blood pressure.

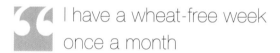
I have a wheat-free week once a month

Why it works: Wheat itself is not necessarily the devil; it's just that Western diets are overloaded with wheat products, which can lead to intolerance. Bloating, flatulence and tiredness are some of the signs of a slight intolerance, so replacing wheat with oats and rye for a week can reduce the chances.

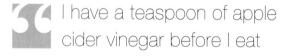
I have a teaspoon of apple cider vinegar before I eat

Why it works: A couple of trials indicate that taking this vinegar before a meal creates a feeling of fullness, thus reducing the amount of food consumed. It can also aid digestion. But it is definitely an acquired taste!

‘I drink chilled green tea mixed with fresh fruit juice and sparkling water when hunger strikes’

Why it works: We often confuse hunger with thirst. A glass of water can take the edge off our hunger, but water can be unexciting. Caffeine-rich green tea mixed with deliciously sweet, vitamin-rich fresh fruit juice and topped up with fizzy water is a great idea. A filling, fat-burning and more exciting solution when water just isn't enough!

 I double the size of my healthy snacks in the week before my period

Why it works: Oestrogen levels are at their lowest and PMS is in full swing at this time of the month, triggering blood sugar fluctuations that make cravings hard to manage. Small and often is the way to go. Increasing the size of your healthy snacks may work for some, having more regular, but smaller healthy snacks may work for others – experiment and find what works for you.

 I write down how I feel after I have eaten

Why it works: This is a great tactic. Some foods make us feel lethargic and low, others give us energy. Uncovering your list of positive foods allows you to get them into your day wherever possible, while avoiding their negative counterparts.

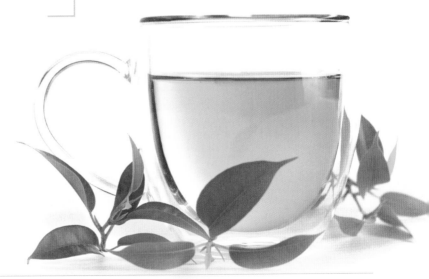

A few more tactics to consider...

— When you keep it simple in the early stages, you're more likely to stick to your plan.

— Every time you find yourself making excuses (e.g. too tired to exercise, no time to cook) note them down somewhere then try to avoid those circumstances in the future.

— Going to bed an hour earlier and getting up an hour earlier means you are not tempted to eat late at night and you have time to exercise first thing in the morning.

— Goal setting is one of the greatest success strategies. Write them down on post-it notes and stick them on the fridge or bathroom mirror, or record them on your mobile phone, and keep referring back to them.

Wearing a pedometer when out walking or jogging has been shown to result in people walking around a mile a day more than those who don't.

— Eating on the run or in a rush creates stress within the body and turns on the fat-storing mechanisms, so take your time when you have the time.

— Having a protein shake can quickly satisfy hunger when your day is full-on. Don't regard them as meal replacements, however, and check the label, as many are loaded with sugar.

— Posting your diet on the internet and sharing your successes and concerns with others works for some. However, be careful: you may end up more confused than when you started!

— Putting money in a jar/box every time you stick to your daily goal means you can afford to give yourself a reward from time to time – preferably not food!

— When you go to the supermarket, park in the far corner of the car park so you have further to walk to and from the store (and the heavier the shopping bags, the more muscle you build!)

— When parking in a multi-storey car park, go straight up to the top level and take the stairs both ways.

— When you take the kids to the park, don't just stand and watch them, go on the swings or run around like they do.

— If you have a dog, try to walk it at the dog's pace rather than training it to walk at yours.

— Don't take the lift unless you have loads to carry. Even if you live or work on the top floor, take the stairs for at least two or three floors then the lift for the remainder (and never take the lift down unless you are in a frantic rush).

— Don't keep biscuits, crisps, pastries or other such foods in the house. If you really, really need a treat, walk to the local shops to get it – at least you're getting some extra exercise!

— Have more sex! Not only is it great at fighting stress, but it burns up the calories (the more energetic it is, the more calories you burn; around 6-7kcals per minute is believed to be the average).

Super supplements

here are a number of nutritional supplements that have been found, in conjunction with diet and lifestyle changes, to encourage fat loss. We've listed some of them below.

However, do remember while they have shown encouraging results in a few studies, research is still in its infancy. In an effort to determine whether there may be one that can help burn fat more efficiently, the overriding recommendation is to consult a health professional.

There are many reasons why using supplementation as any kind of fat-loss accelerator may or may not work, and self medication is not the way to go. It's all too easy to confuse your metabolism and not only will you slow down fat-loss, but you could find yourself a great deal lighter of pocket.

Conjugated linoleic acid (CLA) A growing body of research in the US and Europe shows that CLA reduces body fat and increases lean tissue.

Chromium Preliminary research in animals and humans suggests that chromium picolinate may increase fat loss by helping to maintain healthy blood sugar levels and curb cravings.

Hydroxycitric acid (HCA) Animal research indicates that HCA can suppress appetite and induce fat loss when taken before meals.

L-carnitine Preliminary studies suggest l-carnitine may be beneficial for fat loss when taken on a long-term basis in combination with regular exercise.

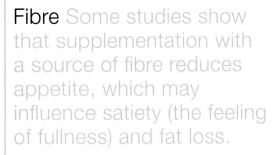

Fibre Some studies show that supplementation with a source of fibre reduces appetite, which may influence satiety (the feeling of fullness) and fat loss.

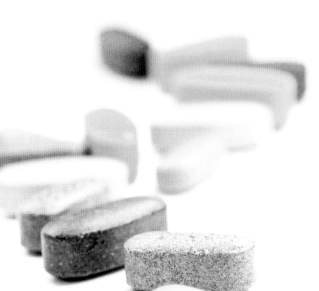

Spirulina This health food is thought to nourish the thyroid gland, which can be underactive in overweight people.

5-HTP An amino acid that may play a role in raising serotonin levels, which in turn reduces appetite.

7-Keto This supplement is believed to raise levels of T3, a thyroid hormone that plays a major role in metabolic rate.

Pyruvate It has been noted that this compound could raise metabolic rate during the metabolism of protein and carbohydrate.

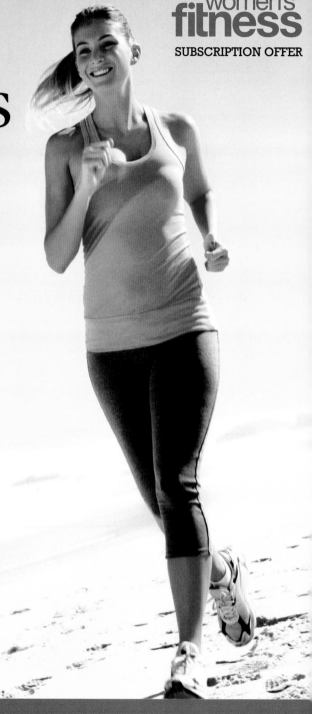

Special offer!

Try 3 issues for just £1

women's fitness
SUBSCRIPTION OFFER

3 ISSUES FOR £1
If you want to learn how to fit regular excerise into your hectic routine without resorting to crash diets, extreme exercise plans or long, exhausting workouts, then *Women's Fitness* is the magazine for you.

SUBSCRIBE TODAY & RECEIVE:
☑ Your first **3 issues for £1**
☑ **28% saving** on all subsequent issues
☑ **FREE delivery** direct to your door
☑ **Inspiring and motivating** to get you moving and staying active.

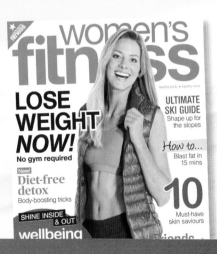

Order online at **www.dennismags.co.uk/womensfitness** or
CALL 0844 844 0246
using offer code: **G1112DP2**

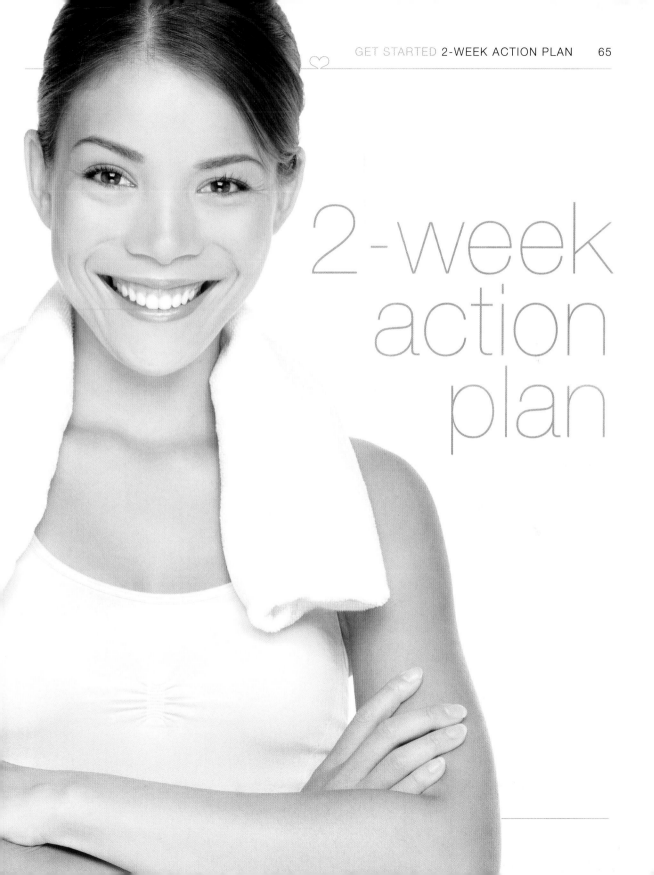

2-week action plan

Time for action!

Spend two weeks in the fast lane to supercharge your fat-burning success

Repetition may work for learning French verbs, but not for successful fat loss. When a diet is too repetitive, boredom quickly kicks in; we feel deprived, start to obsess about food, and cravings invade our day. *The Ultimate 2-Week Fat Loss Diet* offers plenty of variety, so experiment with the choices on offer and find the ones that fit your tastes and priorities. This way, boredom doesn't become an issue.

The golden rules

The following points are an integral part of this energising, mood-boosting, fast-fat-burning plan:

— You have to make it a priority
— You have to eat something every two to three hours
— You have to start it on any day of the week other than a Monday
— You have to bin white foods and only include starchy carbohydrates before 6pm
— You have to fit half an hour's physical activity into your day
— You have to drink water every two to three hours
— You have to keep it simple

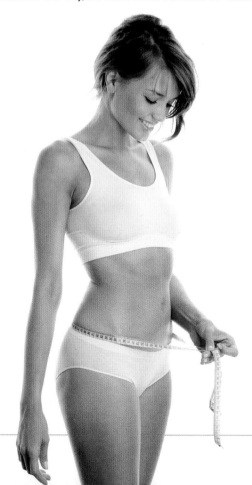

Why should you make it a priority?
Convincing your body to use fat stores for energy in super-quick time requires careful manipulation of the types of foods you eat, so you have to treat it as a project and focus on it.

Why should you eat something every two to three hours?
To keep the fat-burning furnace firing all day, every day, and to avoid energy dips and cravings. When you are tired and hungry, resolve takes a dive.

Why should you start on any day other than Monday?
Successful dieters agree that when you start a diet on a Monday, you see the weekend before as a chance to pig out before the deprivation starts – hardly a recipe for success. Also, you may have noticed that Monday is the only day that seems to attract negative adjectives like 'blue', 'gloomy' and 'depressing'. Why risk it? Plan and shop at the beginning of the week and start midweek.

Why should you bin the white foods?
They are an instant but short-lived energy source, provide few nutrients and don't fill you up for long. They raise the level of glucose in the bloodstream too quickly and, in an effort to get back into balance, sugars are shipped off for immediate use or stored in the liver, muscles and fat cells until required. If you want the fat cells to shrink, you can't afford to give them the chance to expand their storage facilities. They have to be badgered into releasing their stores to provide energy. Keeping your sugar levels balanced by eating colourful, nutrient-rich foods can help to achieve this; white foods make it a whole lot harder.

Why should you avoid eating starchy carbohydrates after 6pm?
Because they provide energy during the day when you are active, but can leave you feeling bloated and uncomfortable at bedtime. It has also been suggested that they promote fat storage through the night (the jury is still out on this one at time of publication, but why risk it?).

Why should you get half an hour's physical activity into your day?
Because working muscles need lots of energy (20-50 times more than they do at rest) so the fat stores are forced into action yet again. And if you get physical first thing in the morning, you fat burn more efficiently for as long as eight hours afterwards (some suggest it may even be 24 hours).

Why should you keep it simple?
Contrary to the spin surrounding some diets, losing fat is not easy, effortless or carefree. You have to commit. While the debate rages on, many successful dieters agree that too much choice can be a major stumbling block in the early stages. That's why we've taken the hard work out of it and provided you with a two-week plan full of delicious and nourishing meals. All you have to do is stick to it!

Why should you drink water every two to three hours?
Because every chemical reaction that takes place in the body, from extracting essential nutrients from food to encouraging fat burning, needs water to produce a result.

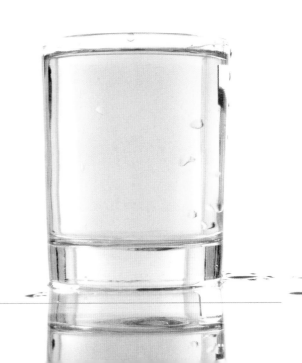

Your daily routine

Follow these steps to burn fat all day long:

1 Get up half an hour earlier, have a small, rich coffee and get physical for 30 minutes.
2 Skin brush before your shower.
3 Eat fruit and drink only juiced fruit/smoothies and still or sparkling water until late morning.
4 Have a late-morning snack.
5 If you need a hot drink, have fresh black coffee or black, green, redbush or herbal/fruit tea before or after your late-morning snack, without milk or sugar.
6 Have soup and salad around lunchtime.
7 If you need another hot drink, choose one of the recommendations above (but not fruit tea).
8 Have a mid-afternoon snack.
9 Have a light meal around dinner time, with no starchy carbohydrates.
10 Have a small bedtime snack at least 30 minutes before you go to bed (only if you are really hungry or you find you are waking up in the early hours and can't get back to sleep).

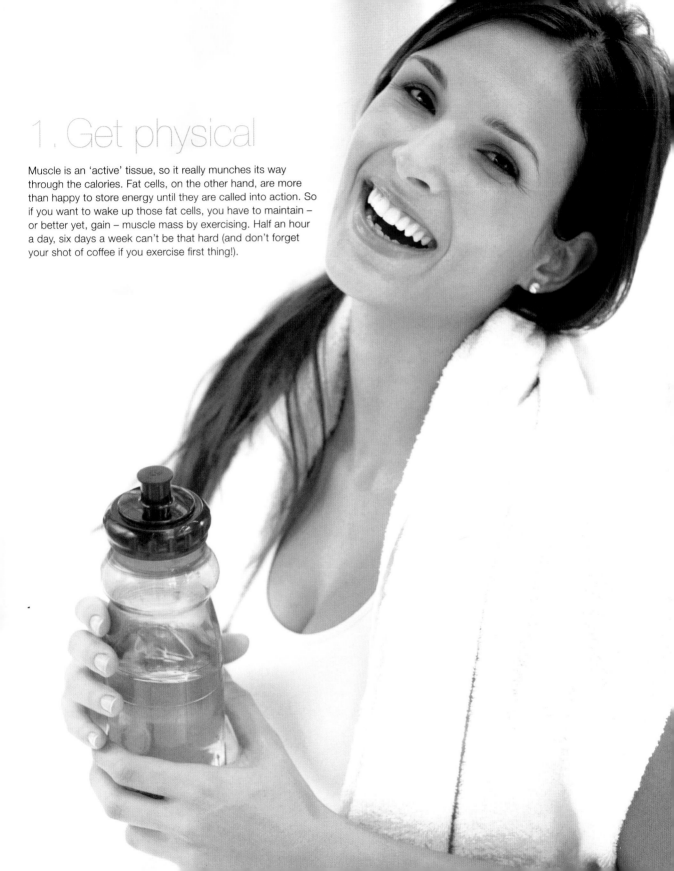

1. Get physical

Muscle is an 'active' tissue, so it really munches its way through the calories. Fat cells, on the other hand, are more than happy to store energy until they are called into action. So if you want to wake up those fat cells, you have to maintain – or better yet, gain – muscle mass by exercising. Half an hour a day, six days a week can't be that hard (and don't forget your shot of coffee if you exercise first thing!).

2. Skin brush

Lightly brushing the skin with a dry brush or loofah stimulates the circulation, removes dead skin cells and promotes the elimination of toxins. Start brushing at your feet and brush towards the heart, then brush from the fingertips up to the shoulders and towards the heart (don't forget the soles of your feet and the palms of your hands). Avoid the face and neck and any damaged or bruised skin. Use small strokes and a gentle pressure – you're not brushing the dog. Jump into the shower straight afterwards and have a good rinse to get rid of the dead skin cells before soaping.

3. Get fruity

A sluggish or inefficient digestive system is one of the most common obstacles to fat loss. Fruit provides a quick energy source and is bursting with nourishment, but when eaten with other foods they can cause havoc for some. If they are trapped in the stomach for too long they ferment, which can not only upset the digestion of other foods but also reduces the nutritional value of the fruit.

When you eat them on their own and on an empty stomach, fruits take a mere 30 minutes to pass through the stomach and, while reaping all their cleansing and nourishing benefits, you avoid the bloating, flatulence or intestinal irritation that you may be all too familiar with.

After your 30 minutes of exercise and every hour thereafter through to late morning (11.30am/noon) have fresh fruit, juiced fruits and fresh fruit smoothies. Go for plenty of variety and wait until late morning before you have your regular cup of tea or coffee.

Select from any of the following, making sure you don't add any proteins or fats (watch out for yoghurt in shop-bought smoothies):

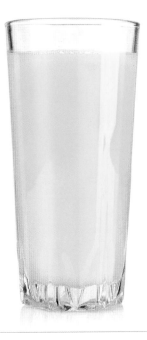

Fresh fruits

Keep the peel on where possible and give them a good scrub before eating whole or chopping, slicing or dicing. Aim for as much colour as possible throughout the morning and be generous with your portions.

Fresh fruit juices

Citrus fruits are made to be juiced. Halve a few oranges and get as much as you can out of them (an electric or battery-operated citrus press is a cheap and highly effective bonus here). Add lemon, lime, mandarin, tangerine, clementine and grapefruit to the mix to ring the changes.

Smoothies

All you need is a blender and you're good to go. Sling a few ice cubes and a teacup of water into the blender, then add fruits of your choice. Berries, cherries (if you can be bothered to stone them), melon, peaches and nectarines, kiwi, tropical fruits like mango, papaya, pineapple and passion fruit, bananas, apples, pears, apricots, plums, grapes, figs, tomatoes (yes, they are a fruit) and, of course, citrus fruits, all blend well. See our quick-fix fruits on page 100 for delicious combinations.

Bags of frozen fruits are great for smoothies if you don't have time to chop, peel and slice. Strain the smoothie through a sieve before drinking if you don't like the seedy/gritty bits and add more water if it's too thick and gloopy. Don't down your smoothie in one go, sip it slowly and savour the flavours.

Juices

If you own a juicer, get it out of the cupboard and go for it. You lose less of the goodness of the fruits (vitamins, minerals and fibre) when you juice them yourself. Pop the juice in a thermos and sip throughout the morning.

Bottled juices and smoothies

These provide the least amount of goodness, as they have been processed to allow them a few days' shelf life. But there are plenty out there that have been sympathetically produced to be as fresh as possible. Price is often a good guide – the more expensive they are, the more goodness they retain because they are less processed, but their shelf life is shorter.

4. Have a late-morning snack

Select from the snacks on page 111, or choose one of
the following and stick to the suggested 2-week diet:

— Small pack of raw unsalted nuts (no dried fruit)
— Cold, cooked chicken leg or breast (skin removed), a
  couple of tomatoes and a handful of raw unsalted nuts
— Couple of oatcakes spread with tinned, mashed salmon
  and topped with cucumber slices
— Raw baby vegetables with a small pot of houmous
— Raw baby vegetables with a small pot of guacamole
— Bowl of mixed olives with feta cheese cubes or olives
  stuffed with anchovies or almonds
— Three-bean salad from the deli section of most
  supermarkets (or make your own)

5. Have a hot drink if you need one

If you usually have coffee or tea in the morning, you may
be struggling by late morning. Now is the time to have
your cuppa. Choose good quality black coffee from ground
beans, or black, green, redbush or herbal/fruit tea. Drink
it before or after your late morning snack, and don't add
milk or sugar.

Have a soya milk latte with no sugar occasionally if the need
for a milky drink is intense.

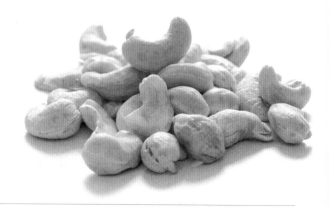

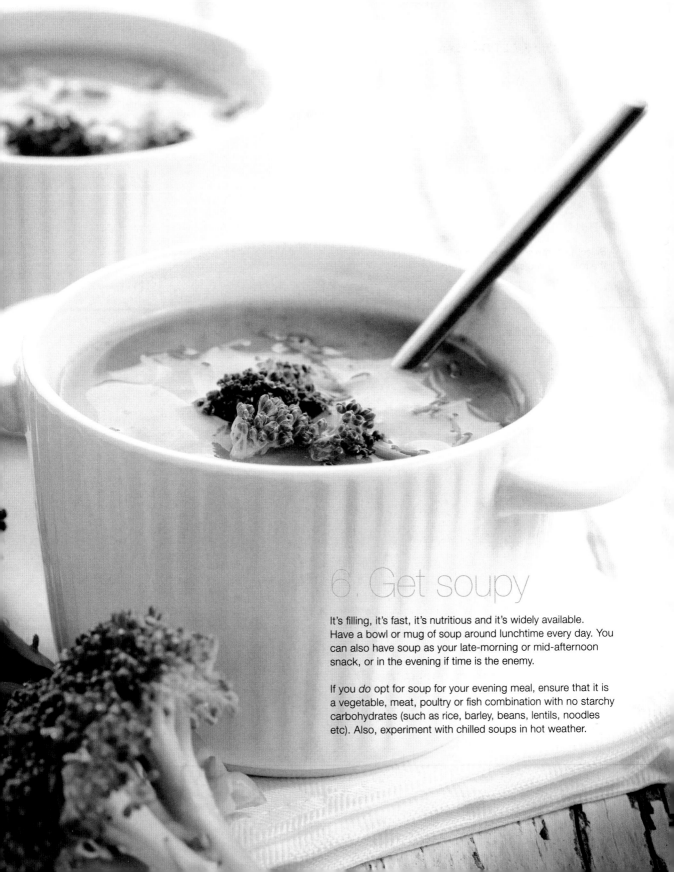

6. Get soupy

It's filling, it's fast, it's nutritious and it's widely available. Have a bowl or mug of soup around lunchtime every day. You can also have soup as your late-morning or mid-afternoon snack, or in the evening if time is the enemy.

If you *do* opt for soup for your evening meal, ensure that it is a vegetable, meat, poultry or fish combination with no starchy carbohydrates (such as rice, barley, beans, lentils, noodles etc). Also, experiment with chilled soups in hot weather.

Home-made soups

If you can find the time, these are the healthiest option as you know exactly what's going into them and you can use as few or as many ingredients as you wish. Experiment with the soups in the recipe section (and remember to leave out the starchy carbohydrates if you are enjoying a bowl after 6pm).

Ready-made soups

There are so many varieties available that you could have three different soups a day, seven days a week for at least a month and never have the same one twice. However, there are a great many that are high in fat, salt or sugar (or all three), so label-reading is vital. Head for the vegetable-y, meaty, fishy, bean-y ones and body swerve the creamy ones (and as before, avoid the ones with starchy carbohydrates after 6pm). Be particularly vigilant about packet and tinned soups. On the label, look at the 'per 100g' column rather than the 'per serving' column and follow these guidelines:

— **Spot the sugar** where it says 'Carbohydrates: of which sugars'; 10g is high, 2g is low. Aim for a maximum of 4g.
— **Spot the saturated fat** where it says 'Fats: of which saturates'; 5g is high, 1g is low. Aim for a maximum of 2g.
— **Spot the salt** where it says 'Salt or salt equivalent'; 1.5g is high, 0.3g is low. Aim for a maximum of 0.6g.
— **Spot the sodium** where it says 'Sodium'; 0.5g is high, 0.1g is low. Aim for a maximum of 0.2g.

Super-quick soups

A spoonful of miso paste or a sachet of miso soup dissolved in boiling water is not only warming and tasty, but it's very nutritious and can keep hunger pangs at bay. Same goes for a mug of Marigold Swiss Vegetable Bouillon. Keep a tub handy and opt for the low-salt version. You can also combine the two.

There are scores of quick soups and cuppa soups on the shelves, but many of them are scarily salt-ridden. Again, check the label. However, if you are following the recommended eating plan and flavouring your food with herbs and spices instead of salt, your salt intake should reduce drastically so your soup choice needn't be the enemy. Just keep an eye on it and follow the salt and sodium guidelines.

Have a small salad

There are lots of suggestions for salads (and dressings) in the recipe section. If you opt for bought/ready-made salads, bin the little pack of salad dressing and replace with a mix of olive, nut or seed oil and a squirt of lemon/lime juice.

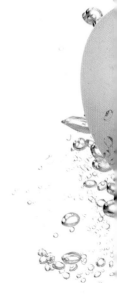

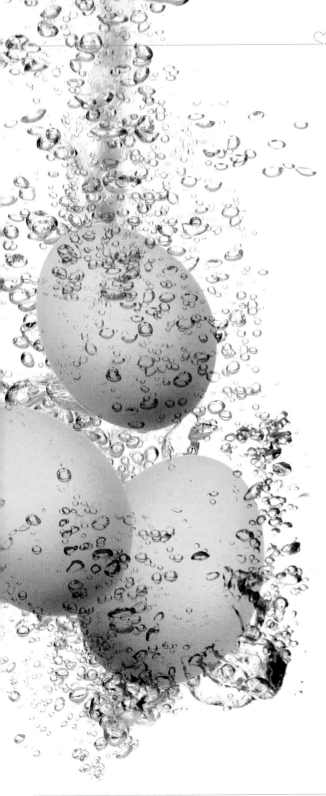

7. Have a hot drink if you need one

Follow the mid-morning recommendations before or after your mid-afternoon snack, but avoid fruit teas.

8. Have a mid-afternoon snack

Select from the snacks on page 111 or choose one of the following to stick to the 2-week diet:

- Small pack of mixed, raw unsalted nuts and seeds (no dried fruit)
- Couple of brown Ryvita with chopped boiled egg mixed with natural live yoghurt and chopped herbs
- Raw baby vegetables with a small pot of cottage cheese
- Raw baby vegetables with a small pot of salsa
- A cold boiled egg and a couple of slices of cooked ham
- A couple of sticks of celery filled with nut butter (almond, cashew, hazelnut, macadamia or peanut)
- A grain bar (go for the ones without dried fruit)

> HOT TIP
> Buy omega-3-rich eggs whenever possible. The hens that lay them are fed on a diet rich in seeds, which provide the essential omega-3 fats that help to promote fat burning. Plus, they taste great!

9. Have a light meal around dinner time

This is the time of the day to say no to starchy carbohydrates. The combination of a decent portion of good quality protein, some essential fats and plenty of vegetables provides a filling meal that gives your body everything it needs to rest, repair and burn fat all night.

You will find light meal suggestions in the 2-week diet and also in the recipe section.

If you are only able to fit your half hour of exercise into the early evening and usually have your meal afterwards, you can add a cupful of brown rice, barley, couscous, beans or lentils, or baked sweet potato.

Have at least three different steamed, grilled, stir-fried or roasted vegetables (not starchy potatoes, root vegetables or corn) and/or a large mixed salad. Top your vegetables or salad with roasted mixed nuts or seeds or mixed beansprouts and drizzle with nut or seed oil (avocado, sesame, sunflower, pumpkin, walnut, linseed, hemp etc) and a squeeze of lemon/lime juice. For ideas, see quick-fix salads (from page 108) and quick-fix vegetables (page 118) in the recipe section.

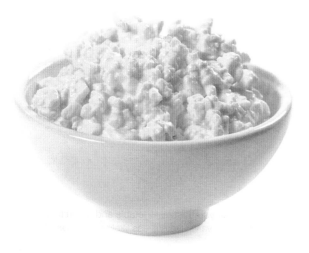

10. Have a bedtime snack

Only do this if you are really hungry, you find you can't get to sleep or if you regularly wake up in the early hours and can't doze off again. The following food combinations are rich in the amino acid tryptophan, which encourages the production of the sleepy chemical, serotonin; plus if your blood sugar is all over the place it can help to get the balance right overnight. Have your snack at least 30 minutes before you go to bed. You will probably find after a few days on the diet you will be sleeping better and it won't be required.

— A couple of mini oatcakes with nut or seed butter and a couple of slices of cold turkey breast
— A mug of Green and Black's dark hot chocolate made with soya milk
— A small tub of natural cottage cheese with a handful of mixed seeds
— One egg, lightly scrambled, on an oatcake.
— A small carton of natural live yoghurt with a swirl of honey
— Two or three squares of dark chocolate (70% cocoa solids minimum) and a few shavings of Parmesan cheese
— A small plate of porridge made with water and topped with a spoonful of manuka honey

It's easy to follow

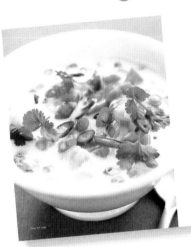

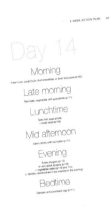

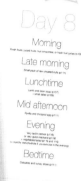

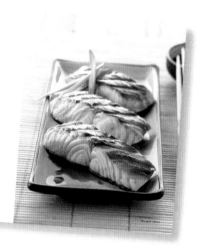

Your 2-week plan starts here

Stick to the plan that follows as closely as possible for two weeks. But don't panic if time is against you and you haven't planned ahead. The quick-fix rescue plan at the back of the book provides shop-bought and on-the-go strategies that won't wreck your diet. Photocopy it and keep it to hand to get you out of trouble.

After two weeks you can continue the plan for as long as you wish, especially if you are the type who prefers to stick fairly rigidly to a regime. Or, you can play around with the recipe/snack suggestions (and the quick-fix rescue plan strategies) to suit your tastes, timetable and commitments. If you keep things varied you're less likely to get bored!

Remember:

- Eat only fruit until 11.30am/noon.
- Have a bowl of soup at lunchtime.
- Have a creative mix of salad stuffs with your soup (see salad suggestions on page 108).
- Avoid starchy carbohydrates after 6pm (no rice, pasta, bread, potatoes, sweet potatoes, beans, lentils, root vegetables or corn). See carbohydrate choices on page 98 if you exercise in the evening.
- Have at least three vegetables or a big salad with your evening meal (see salad suggestions on page 110 and vegetable suggestions on page 119).
- Have a bedtime snack only if you are really hungry or sleep is a struggle.
- Swap mid-morning and mid-afternoon snacks around freely or just concentrate on the ones you like best (see snacks on page 111 for full list).
- Get back on track as quickly as you can if things go awry, it was merely a blip!

First thing in the morning
- Double espresso (no milk or sugar).
- 30 minutes' exercise followed by a large glass of water.
- Skin brush and shower.

Every hour until late morning
(11.30am/noon)
- Fresh fruits, juiced fruits, fruit smoothies and fresh fruit juices.

Late morning and mid afternoon
- Hot drink.

Throughout the day
(Every couple of hours)
- Still or sparkling water.

Day 1

Morning

Fresh fruits; fruit smoothies; or fresh fruit juices (p100)

Late morning

Small pack of raw unsalted nuts

Lunchtime

Beef broth with pearl barley (p104)
+ small salad (p108)

Mid afternoon

Ryvita and chopped egg (p111)

Evening

Fish fillets Thai-style (p114)
or very quick salmon (p116)
+ vegetables/salad (p119 and p110)
(+ starchy carbohydrate if you exercise in the evening)

Bedtime

Oatcakes and turkey slices (p111)

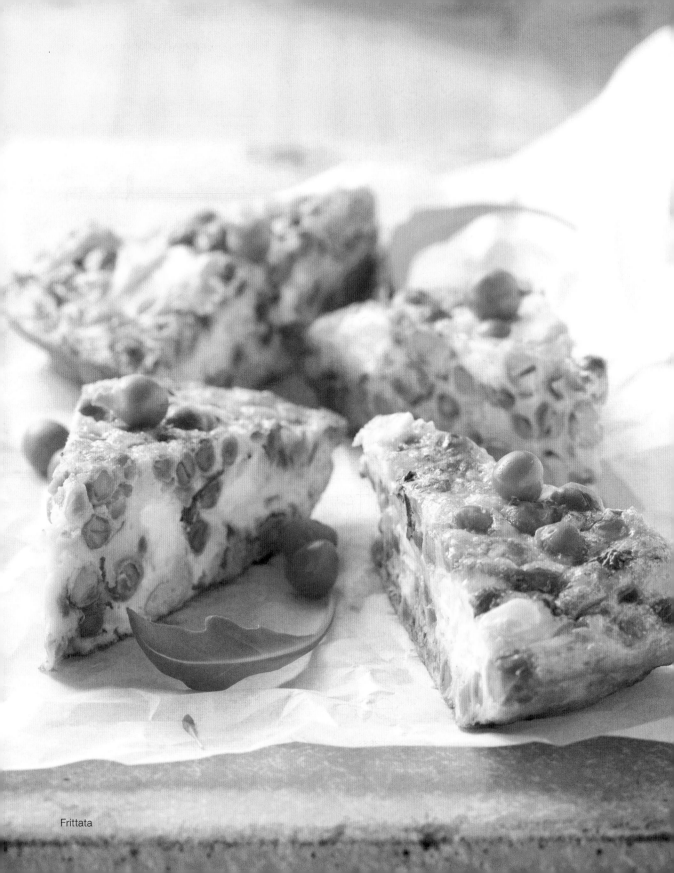

Frittata

Day 2

Morning

Fresh fruits; juiced fruits; fruit smoothies; or fresh fruit juices (p100)

Late morning

Oatcakes with tinned salmon and cucumber (p111)

Lunchtime

Spicy pepper and sweet potato soup (p105)
+ small salad (p108)

Mid afternoon

Grain bar (p111)

Evening

Frittata (p113)
or very quick omelette (p116)
+ vegetables/salad (p119 and 110)
(+ starchy carbohydrate if you exercise in the evening)

Bedtime

Cottage cheese and seeds (p111)

Day 3

Morning

Fresh fruits; juiced fruits; fruit smoothies; or fresh fruit juices (p100)

Late morning

Raw baby vegetables with houmous (p111)

Lunchtime

Chinese little gem and chicken/tofu soup (p102)
+ small salad (p108)

Mid afternoon

Cold boiled egg and ham (p111)

Evening

Tomato, squah and spinach curry (p114)
or very quick mackerel (p118)
+ vegetables/salad (p119 and 110)
(+ starchy carbohydrate if you exercise in the evening)

Bedtime

Porridge and honey (p111)

Day 4

Morning

Fresh fruits; juiced fruits; fruit smoothies; or fresh fruit juices (p100)

Late Morning

Cold cooked chicken, tomatoes and raw unsalted nuts (p111)

Lunchtime

Lentil soup (p107)
+ small salad (p108)

Mid Afternoon

Raw baby vegetables with salsa (p111)

Evening

Very quick prawns (p118)
or very quick fish (p116)
+ vegetables/salad (p119 and 110)
(+ starchy carbohydrate if you exercise in the evening)

Bedtime

Dark chocolate and cheese (p111)

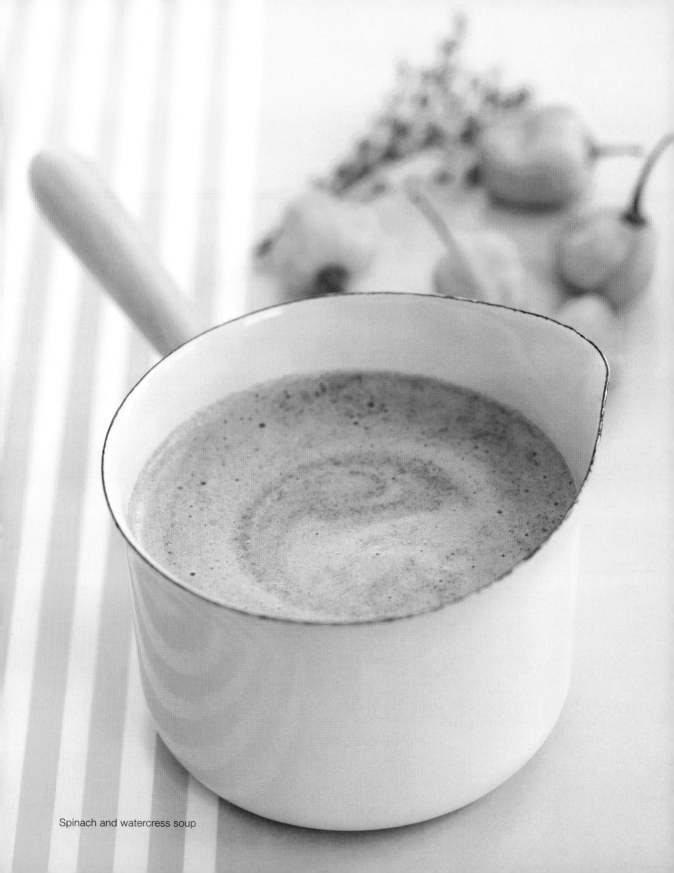

Spinach and watercress soup

Day 5

Morning

Fresh fruits; juiced fruits; fruit smoothies; or fresh fruit juices (p100)

Late morning

Three-bean salad (p111)

Lunchtime

Spinach and watercress soup (p107)
+ small salad (p108)

Mid afternoon

Raw baby vegetables with cottage cheese (p111)

Evening

Beef stew (p112)
or very quick chicken (p116)
+ vegetables/salad (p119 and 110)
(+ starchy carbohydrate if you exercise in the evening)

Bedtime

Yoghurt and honey (p111)

Day 6

Morning

Fresh fruits; juiced fruits; fruit smoothies; or fresh fruit juices (p100)

Late morning

Mixed olives with feta cheese or stuffed olives (p111)

Lunchtime

Spicy red lentil soup (p105)
+ small salad (p108)

Mid afternoon

Small pack of raw unsalted nuts and seeds (p111)

Evening

Very quick pork (p118)
or very quick lamb (p118)
+ vegetables/salad (p119 and 110)
(+ starchy carbohydrate if you exercise in the evening)

Bedtime

Cottage cheese and seeds (p111)

Day 7

Morning

Fresh fruits; juiced fruits; fruit smoothies; or fresh fruit juices (p100)

Late morning

Raw baby vegetables with guacamole (p111)

Lunchtime

Chicken and vegetable soup (p102)
+ small salad (p108)

Mid afternoon

Celery sticks with nut butter (p111)

Evening

Turkey burgers (p112)
or very quick burgers (p118)
+ vegetables/salad (p119 and 110)
(+ starchy carbohydrate if you exercise in the evening)

Bedtime

Oatcake and scrambled egg (p111)

Day 8

Morning

Fresh fruits; juiced fruits; fruit smoothies; or fresh fruit juices (p100)

Late morning

Small pack of raw unsalted nuts (p111)

Lunchtime

Lamb and bean soup (p107)
+ small salad (p108)

Mid afternoon

Ryvita and chopped egg (p111)

Evening

Very quick salmon (p116)
or very quick mackerel (p118)
+ vegetables/salad (p119 and 110)
(+ starchy carbohydrate if you exercise in the evening)

Bedtime

Oatcakes and turkey slices (p111)

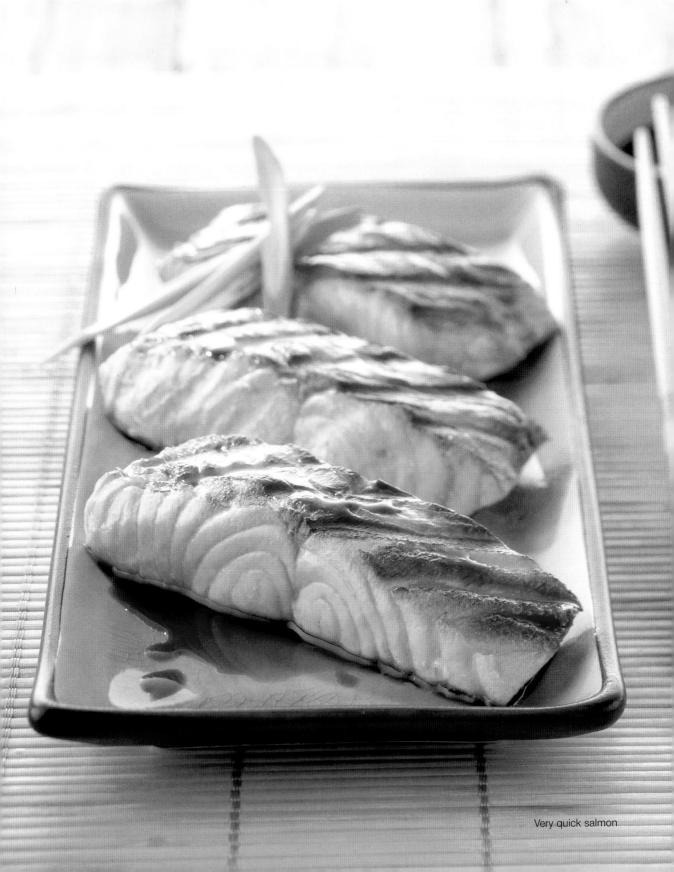

Very quick salmon

Day 9

Morning

Fresh fruits; juiced fruits; fruit smoothies; or fresh fruit juices (p100)

Late morning

Oatcakes with tinned salmon and cucumber (p111)

Lunchtime

Pea, mint and lettuce soup (p104)
+ small salad (p108)

Mid afternoon

Grain bar (p111)

Evening

Very quick omelette (p116)
or frittata (p113)
+ vegetables/salad (p119 and 110)
(+ starchy carbohydrate if you exercise in the evening)

Bedtime

Yoghurt and honey (p111)

Day 10

Morning

Fresh fruits; juiced fruits; fruit smoothies; or fresh fruit juices (p100)

Late morning

Raw baby vegetables with houmous (p111)

Lunchtime

Chicken and vegetable soup (p102)
+ small salad (p108)

Mid afternoon

Cold boiled egg and ham (p111)

Evening

Tomato, squash and spinach curry (p114)
or very quick pork (p118)
+ vegetables/salad (p119 and 110)
(+ starchy carbohydrate if you exercise in the evening)

Bedtime

Porridge and honey (p111)

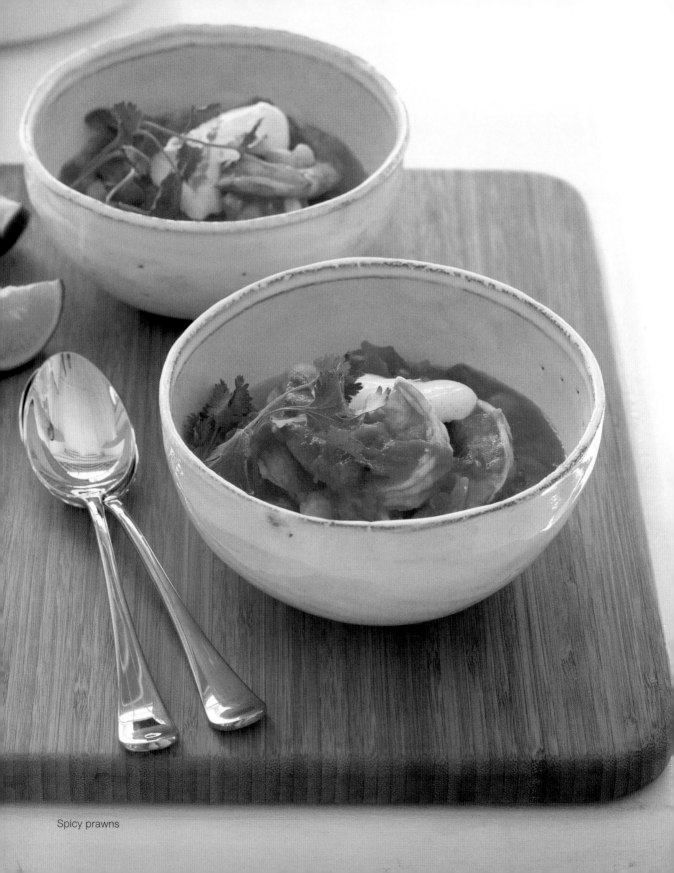

Spicy prawns

Day 11

Morning

Fresh fruits; juiced fruits; fruit smoothies; or fresh fruit juices (p100)

Late morning

Cold cooked chicken, tomatoes and raw unsalted nuts (p111)

Lunchtime

Lamb and bean soup (p107)
+ small salad (p108)

Mid afternoon

Raw baby vegetables with salsa (p111)

Evening

Spicy prawns (p113)
or very quick fish (p116)
+ vegetables/salad (pages 119 and 110)
(+ starchy carbohydrate if you exercise in the evening)

Bedtime

Dark chocolate and cheese (p111)

Day 12

Morning

Fresh fruits; juiced fruits; fruit smoothies; or fresh fruit juices (p100)

Late morning

Three-bean salad (p111)

Lunchtime

Long-stemmed broccoli soup (p105)
+ small salad (p108)

Mid afternoon

Raw baby vegetables with cottage cheese (p111)

Evening

Very quick lamb (p118)
or very quick tofu (p118)
+ vegetables/salad (p119 and 110)
(+ starchy carbohydrate if you exercise in the evening)

Bedtime

Yoghurt and honey (p111)

Day 13

Morning

Fresh fruits; juiced fruits; fruit smoothies; or fresh fruit juices (p100)

Late morning

Mixed olives with feta cheese or stuffed olives (p111)

Lunchtime

Spicy red pepper and sweet potato soup (p105)
+ small salad (p108)

Mid afternoon

Small pack of raw unsalted nuts and seeds (p111)

Evening

Beef stroganoff (p114)
or very quick chicken (p116)
+ vegetables/salad (p119 and 110)
(+ starchy carbohydrate if you exercise in the evening)

Bedtime

Cottage cheese and seeds (p111)

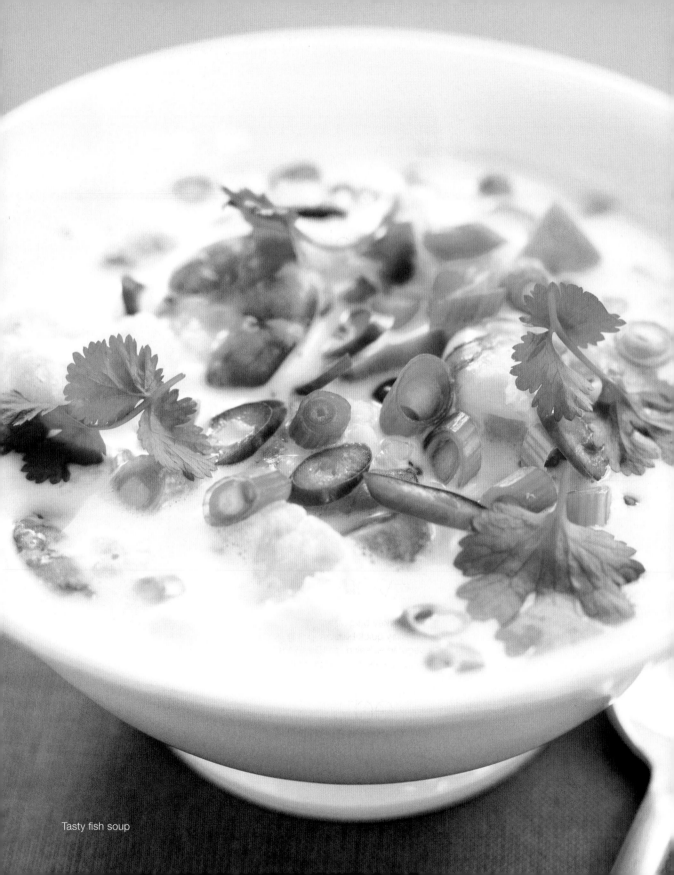

Tasty fish soup

Day 14

Morning

Fresh fruits; juiced fruits; fruit smoothies; or fresh fruit juices (p100)

Late morning

Raw baby vegetables with guacamole (p111)

Lunchtime

Tasty fish soup (p104)
+ small salad (p108)

Mid afternoon

Celery sticks with nut butter (p111)

Evening

Turkey burgers (p112)
or very quick burgers (p118)
+ vegetables/salad (p119 and 110)
(+ starchy carbohydrate if you exercise in the evening)

Bedtime

Oatcake and scrambled egg (p111)

Post-exercise treats

Choose from these starchy carbohydrate choices to include if you exercise in the evening (or have an action-packed night ahead!)

– cup of quick-cook couscous
– cup of quick-cook brown rice
– cup of quick-cook quinoa
– cup of tinned, cooked beans (kidney, haricot, black-eyed, borlotti, cannellini, flageolet, broad beans, chickpeas or mixed)
– cup of tinned, cooked lentils (red, green, Puy or mixed)
– small baked sweet potato
– baked sweet potato chips (cut a small sweet potato into chips, drizzle with a little olive oil, put on a roasting tray in a hot oven and bake until cooked through and crispy outside)

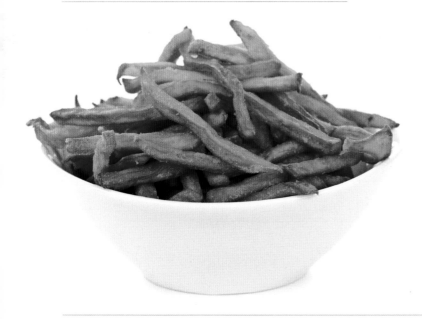

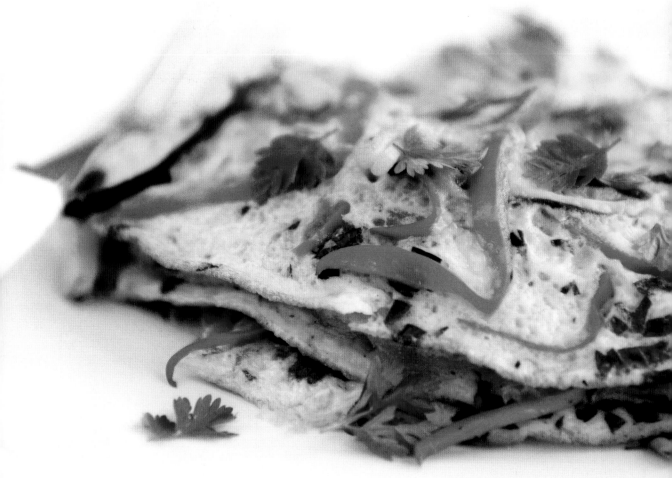

Fat-burning recipes

Quick and easy meals to help you slim

Juices & smoothies

A quick and healthy way to get your five-a-day

Less is definitely more when it comes to fruit drinks. It is tempting to throw in every tired-looking specimen that is lurking in the fruit bowl, and the desire to sling in half a banana to give a bit more substance can kill many a good smoothie. A delicious, satisfying fruit drink relies on just a few ingredients, but combination is key.

Get the blender out, sling in a few ice cubes and a teacup of cold water then add your fruits of choice, chopped into bite-sized pieces (remember to keep the skin on and just give them a good scrub, wherever possible).

Whizz slowly at first until the ingredients start to come together, then go for maximum power until smooth. Add the extras (fruit juice/herbs/spices/flavourings) then blitz again briefly. Add cold water if you need to thin it down, strain the juice through a sieve if you don't like the seedy/gritty bits and sip slowly while you rinse out the blender. Put any extra in a flask for later in the morning.

Here are a few winning combinations that take a maximum of five minutes:

— Apple and blueberry with fresh lemon juice and cinnamon
— Apple, raspberry and grapes with fresh orange juice
— Apple and plum with morello cherry juice and a drizzle of honey
— Grapefruit, passion fruit and pineapple
— Tangerine, strawberry and banana
— Mango and mixed berries with fresh lime juice
— Watermelon and cantaloupe melon with cold green tea
— Rhubarb, orange, fresh ginger and mint leaves
— Peach, raspberry and redcurrants with rose water
— Pear, melon and blackberries with ground black pepper
— Tomato, orange and apple with fresh basil

These combinations feature fresh fruits, but the whole exercise can become even swifter if you have a few bags of frozen fruits in the freezer. Try tropical fruit mixes, summer berry mixes, rhubarb, cranberries, blueberries, blackberries, blackcurrants, redcurrants and pineapples. You can use them straight from the freezer, which means you can dispense with the ice cubes.

Other fresh juices, herbs, spices and flavourings you might like to add to your fruit selection include: apple, pineapple, passion fruit, cranberry or grapefruit juice; fresh oregano, lemon thyme or spearmint, grated nutmeg or powdered allspice; vanilla essence and balsamic or fruit vinegars.

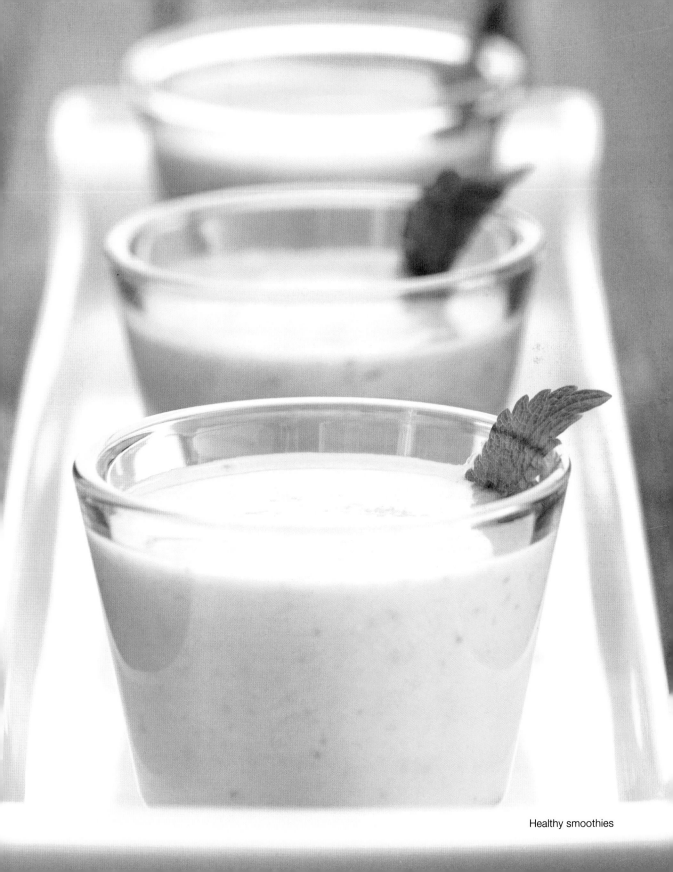

Healthy smoothies

Healthy filling soups

Ward off hunger with quick tasty soups

Chinese little gem & chicken/tofu soup

Prep and cook time: 35 mins

Ingredients: (for 2 servings)
1tbsp olive oil
1 small clove garlic, crushed
2cm piece of fresh ginger, crushed
6 spring onions, white part chopped finely, green part cut into 5cm pieces
2tsp Marigold Vegetable Bouillon powder in 500ml hot water
2 small chicken breasts finely sliced along the grain of the chicken and/or 50g tofu, cubed
1 small carrot, finely sliced
1 stick celery, finely sliced
1 little gem lettuce, finely sliced
Good splash of light soya sauce

Method:
1 Warm the oil, add the garlic, ginger and white spring onion and sauté for 2 mins.
2 Add the stock and bring to a simmer, add the chicken and/ or tofu, green part of the spring onion, carrot, celery, lettuce and soya sauce and cook gently for 5 mins before serving.

Bok Choy is a good substitute for the lettuce and if you want to bulk the soup out a bit add a tablespoon of brown rice and cook well in the stock before adding the chicken/ tofu and vegetables.

Chicken and vegetable soup

Prep and cook time: 40 mins

Ingredients: (for 2 servings)
2tsp Marigold Vegetable Bouillon powder in 500ml hot water
2 small skinless chicken breasts
1tbsp olive oil
1 small onion, finely chopped
1 garlic clove, finely chopped
2 small carrots, finely diced
1 celery stick, finely sliced
2tbsp finely chopped fresh parsley
Sea salt and freshly ground black pepper

Method:
1 Bring stock to a simmer in a medium-sized pan.
2 Add chicken and simmer very gently, uncovered for 6 mins.
3 Remove pan from heat, cover and let stand until chicken is cooked through, about 15 mins.
4 Transfer chicken to a plate to cool. Reserve poaching liquid.
5 While chicken is poaching, sauté onion in oil until softened.
6 Add garlic and sauté for a further minute.
7 Add carrots and celery and sauté, covered, stirring occasionally until softened, 8 to 10 mins.
8 Add poaching liquid and simmer, covered until vegetables are tender then remove from heat.
9 While vegetables are cooking, shred chicken and stir into soup just before serving with parsley. Season to taste.

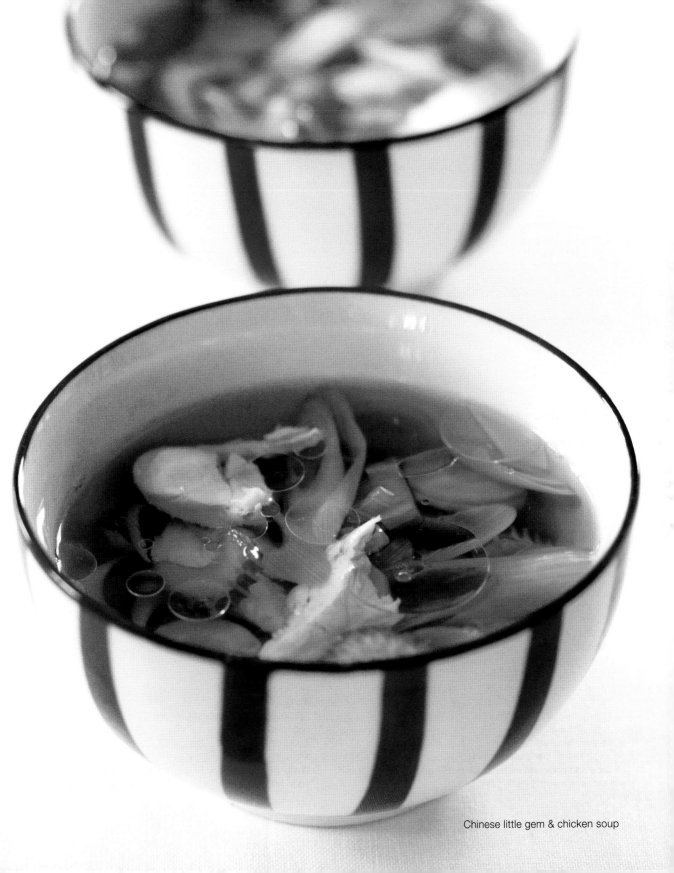

Chinese little gem & chicken soup

Pea, mint and lettuce soup

Prep and cook time: 20 mins

Ingredients: (for 2 servings)
2tsp Marigold Vegetable Bouillon powder in 500ml hot water
250g frozen peas
6 large green lettuce leaves, washed and shredded
Handful fresh mint leaves
Sea salt crystals and freshly ground black pepper

Method:
1 Put the stock in a good-sized pan and bring to the boil. Add peas and simmer until tender (10 mins).
2 Add mint leaves and shredded lettuce and simmer for a couple more minutes.
3 Whizz with a hand blender until smooth and season according to taste.

Tasty fish soup

Prep and cook time: 20 mins

Ingredients: (for 2 servings)
1tbsp light olive oil
1 clove garlic, finely sliced
½tsp peeled, grated fresh ginger
¼tsp red chilli, seeds removed, very finely chopped
1tsp bashed, finely chopped lemongrass (or use ready-chopped from a jar)
200g fresh crab meat (tinned if you are in a rush)
500ml fish stock (most supermarkets have handy tubs)
150ml coconut milk
1tbsp Thai fish sauce, or to taste
50g uncooked shelled de-veined prawns
1 spring onion, finely sliced
Lemon juice, to taste
1tbsp chopped fresh coriander
Freshly ground black pepper

Method:
1 Heat the oil in a large pan over a medium heat then add the garlic, ginger, chilli, lemongrass and crab meat and sauté for 4-5 mins.

2 Pour in the stock, coconut milk and fish sauce, increase the heat to high and bring to the boil.
3 Reduce the heat to low, tip in the prawns and simmer very gently for 1-2 mins, until the prawns are pink and cooked through.
4 Stir in the spring onion, lemon juice and coriander and season to taste.

Beef broth with pearl barley

Prep and cook time: 50 mins

Ingredients: (for 2 servings)
1tbsp olive oil
250g lean stewing steak, cut into small cubes
2tsp balsamic vinegar
2tsp Worcestershire sauce
1 small onion, finely chopped
1 carrot, finely diced
1 stick celery, finely sliced
1 small bay leaf
1 small sprig fresh rosemary
2tsp Marigold Vegetable Bouillon powder in 500ml hot water
75g pearl barley
Handful chopped fresh parsley
Sea salt and freshly ground black pepper

Method:
1 Warm the oil in a medium-sized pan and gently brown the meat over a medium heat.
2 Add the balsamic vinegar and Worcestershire sauce, turn up the heat and stir vigorously until most of the liquid has been absorbed.
3 Add the vegetables, bay leaf and rosemary, put the lid on and cook over a low heat until vegetables are tender, about 20 mins.
4 Add the stock and bring to the boil.
5 Add pearl barley and parsley and simmer until the barley is tender (25 mins).
6 Take the pan off the heat and remove the bay leaf and rosemary. Season to taste.
7 Whizz with a hand blender to preferred texture. Add boiling water to thin if necessary.

Spicy red pepper and sweet potato soup

Prep and cook time: 40 mins

Ingredients: (for 2 servings)
1tbsp olive oil
1 small onion, finely sliced
1 small garlic clove, crushed
1 stick celery, finely sliced
1 small (or ½ large) red pepper, de-seeded and finely sliced
1 small (or ½ large) yellow pepper, de-seeded and finely sliced
1 small (or ½ large) orange pepper, de-seeded and finely sliced
1 small (or ½ large) sweet potato, peeled and finely diced
1 small tin (or ½ large tin) chopped tomatoes
½ fresh chilli or 1tsp powdered chilli
2 tsp Marigold Vegetable Bouillon powder in 500ml hot water
Sea salt and freshly ground black pepper

Method:
1 Warm the olive oil in a medium-sized pan, add all the vegetables and fresh chilli if using and cook over a medium heat until tender.
2 Add the tomatoes, chilli powder (if not using fresh) and vegetable stock.
3 Bring to the boil and simmer for a further 5 mins then mash well to give a chunky texture or blend if you prefer a smooth soup. Season to taste.

Spicy red lentil soup

Prep and cook time: 40 mins

Ingredients: (for 2 servings)
1tsp olive oil
1tsp paprika
1tsp turmeric
Small pinch cinnamon
Small pinch cayenne pepper
1 small onion, finely chopped
1 medium carrot, scrubbed and diced
1 small red pepper, de-seeded and finely chopped
75g red split lentils, rinsed
½ tin chopped tomatoes
2tsp Marigold Vegetable Bouillon powder in 500ml hot water
1tsp dried basil or Italian mixed herbs
1 small bay leaf
Sea salt and freshly ground black pepper

Method:
1 Warm the oil and lightly sauté the spices.
2 Add vegetables and lentils and stir to coat with spices.
3 Add tomatoes, stock, basil and bay leaf.
4 Bring to the boil and simmer for 40 mins or until the lentils and vegetables are cooked.
5 Remove the bay leaf, season to taste and add more water if necessary.

Long-stemmed broccoli soup

Prep and cook time: 30 mins

Ingredients: (for 2 servings)
50g sun-dried tomatoes in oil, roughly chopped (keep oil)
1 small onion, finely sliced
1 clove garlic, finely sliced
Small pinch chilli powder
200g long-stem broccoli, trimmed and roughly sliced
2tsp Marigold Vegetable Bouillon powder in 500ml hot water
Small bunch fresh parsley, finely chopped
Sea salt and freshly ground black pepper
Lemon juice

Method:
1 Heat one tablespoon of the oil from the sun-dried tomatoes and gently sauté the onion until soft.
2 Add the sun-dried tomatoes, garlic and chilli powder half way through and stir frequently. Add the broccoli and continue to toss for a few minutes.
3 Add most of the stock and gently simmer for 10 mins or until the broccoli is tender.
4 Use a hand blender or whizz in a food processor until you have a nice chunky consistency, using the remaining stock or a little boiling water if the soup is too thick.
5 Stir through the parsley, season to taste and add a splash of lemon juice.

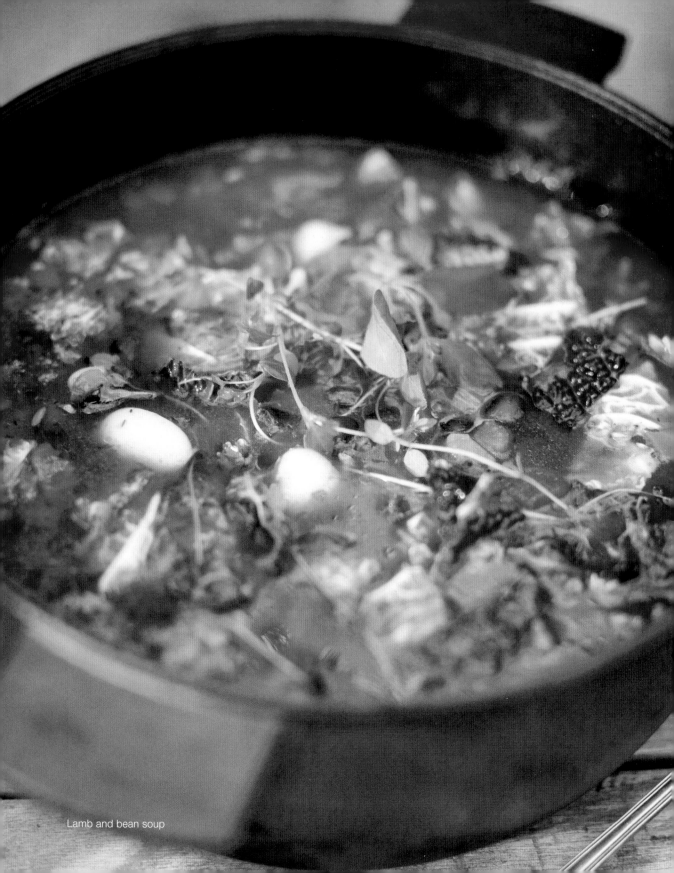

Lamb and bean soup

Lamb and bean soup

Prep and cook time: 40 mins

Ingredients: (for 2 servings)
100g lean lamb mince
½tbsp Worcester sauce
½tsp each of ground cumin, paprika and chilli
1tbsp olive oil
1 small onion, finely chopped
1 clove garlic, finely chopped
1 small red pepper, thinly sliced
1 carrot, sliced into thin strips
½ tin black-eyed or canellini beans, drained (keep the liquid)
1 baby cabbage or 1 little gem lettuce, finely sliced
2 tomatoes, skinned and chopped, or 2 tinned plum tomatoes, chopped
2tsp Marigold Vegetable Bouillon powder in 500ml hot water
Fresh parsley or coriander leaves
Sea salt and freshly ground black pepper

Method:
1 Brown the meat in a non-stick pan, add the Worcestershire sauce and keep stirring until the meat is browned and the liquid is absorbed. Add spices and stir well.
2 Heat the oil in another pan, cook the onion and garlic until soft. Add the pepper and carrot, cook for 5 more minutes.
3 Whizz one third of the beans in a food processor.
4 Add the bean liquid, most of the stock, puréed beans and cabbage (if using) and simmer gently for 15 minutes.
5 Add the tomatoes, remaining beans and lettuce (if not using cabbage) and cook for a further 5 minutes.
6 Add more stock if the soup is too thick.
7 Season and garnish with chopped parsley or coriander.

Spinach and watercress soup

Prep and cook time: 20 mins

Ingredients: (for 2 servings)
1tbsp olive oil
1 small onion, roughly chopped
2tsp Marigold Vegetable Bouillon powder in 500ml

hot water
1 level dessertspoon porridge oats
½ bag fresh spinach
½ bag fresh watercress
Sea salt and freshly ground black pepper
Lemon juice

Method:
1 Warm the oil and sauté onion until soft.
2 Add the stock and porridge, bring to the boil then simmer until porridge is cooked (10-15 minutes).
3 Add spinach and watercress, bring soup back to the boil then use a hand blender until you have a smooth consistency.
4 Season and add lemon juice to taste.

Lentil soup

Prep and cook time: 35 mins

Ingredients: (for 2 servings)
1 thin leek, washed and finely sliced
1 stick celery, finely sliced
2 large carrots, scrubbed and diced
2tsp Marigold Vegetable Bouillon powder in 500ml hot water
75g red split lentils, rinsed
Small bunch curly parsley, finely chopped
Sea salt and freshly ground black pepper

Method:
1 Put leek, celery and carrot into a good-sized pan, add stock and bring to the boil. Turn heat down and add the lentils.
2 Simmer for 20 mins or until the lentils are cooked.
3 Add the parsley then mash to a nice chunky texture or whizz with a hand blender until smooth. Season to taste.

Toppings for soups:
– Pesto; natural yoghurt or tzatziki; salsa; nut or seed oil; Worcestershire sauce, soya sauce or balsamic vinegar; beansprouts; toasted nuts and/or seeds; fresh herbs; dried or powdered spice; grated ginger; diced chilli; chopped tomatoes; diced apple; crispy seaweed or nori flakes; steamed asparagus tips; chopped chives or spring onions.

Satisfying salads

Boost your basic salads with these tips for wholesome lunches and dinners

Lunchtime salads

(starchy carbohydrates can be included)

If you have time to make your own:
Base: All kinds of lettuce, spinach leaves, watercress, rocket, fresh parsley and mixed herbs, sliced fennel, spring onions, sliced red onions, Chinese leaves, bok choy, mustard cress, baby gem lettuce, chicory leaves, celery leaves, chives, shredded cabbage, celery, finely sliced leeks.

Next: Tomatoes (fresh and sun-dried), cucumber, beansprouts, green beans, white beans, red beans, chickpeas, lentils, grated carrot, grated courgettes, radishes, red, yellow and orange peppers, sweetcorn, baby corn, sugar snap peas, mangetouts, mild chillies, peas, sliced avocado, baby asparagus, cold cooked brown rice, couscous, bulgur wheat or quinoa, sliced mushrooms, artichoke hearts, olives, roasted vegetables.

Consider: A little cold cooked skinless chicken or turkey, cold sliced skinless duck or game, a few crispy bacon bits, lean cooked meats, Swiss cheeses (cubed, sliced or grated), feta cheese, goats' cheese, cottage cheese, cooked peeled prawns, flaked mackerel, flaked hot-smoked salmon or trout, anchovies, sardines, fresh or tinned tuna, crab or salmon, sliced or chopped boiled egg or whole quail eggs.

To finish: Slug of extra virgin olive oil or nut/seed oil, lemon or lime juice, balsamic, red or white wine vinegar, sea salt flakes, ground black pepper, soya sauce, fresh nuts (whole, toasted, chopped or flaked), seeds, natural yoghurt or cottage cheese, wholegrain mustard, crushed garlic or ginger, drizzle of honey, spoonful of fruity/spicy chutney or creamed horseradish, spoonful of peanut butter, tahini, houmous or tzatziki, shake of chilli or curry powder, Worcestershire sauce, Tabasco, tomato purée, sprinkling of chopped herbs.

NB: If you are taking a salad to work or out and about, keep the dressing separate and add it just before you eat.

If you are going for shop-bought salads:
Keep all the above guidelines in mind, ensure that leafy greens and fresh vegetables form at least 50 per cent of the mix and if not, bulk the salad out with an extra bag of green leaves and whenever possible bin the little packet of dressing that is often included (they can be loaded with sugar) and add your own oil/lemon juice/vinegar, or do without.

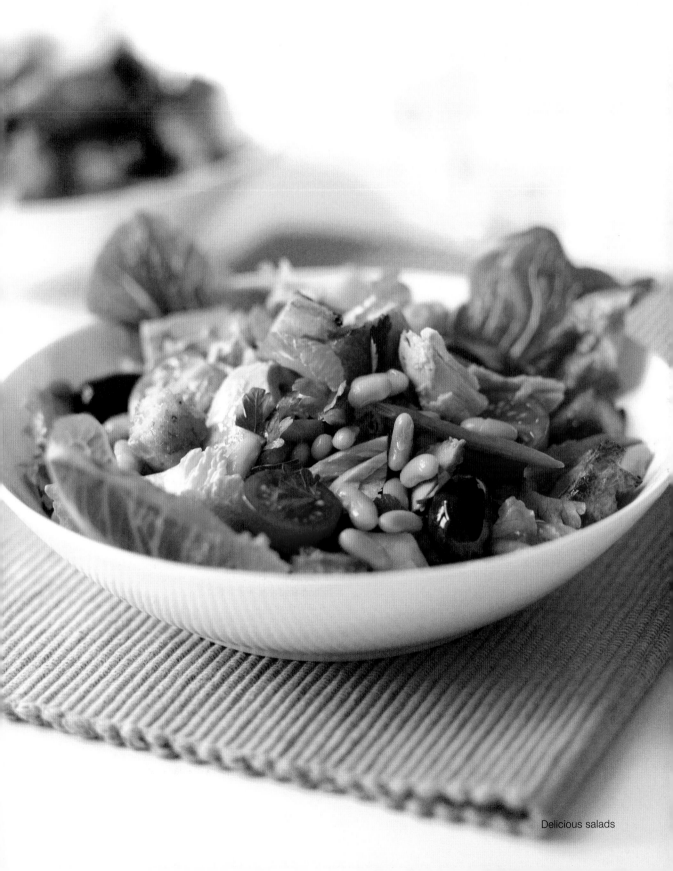

Delicious salads

Salads with your evening meal

(no starchy carbohydrates included)

When having a salad either with your dinner or as your evening meal, really fill your plate with greens and colourful veggies. If the salad is your main meal, be sure to include protein too. Remember not to include any starchy carbohydrates in evening salads.

If you have time to make your own:
Base: All kinds of lettuce, spinach leaves, watercress, rocket, fresh parsley and mixed herbs, sliced fennel, spring onions, sliced red onions, Chinese leaves, bok choy, mustard cress, baby gem lettuce, chicory leaves, celery leaves, chives, shredded cabbage, celery, finely sliced leeks.

Next: Tomatoes (fresh and sun-dried), cucumber, beansprouts, green beans, grated carrot, grated courgettes, radishes, red, yellow and orange peppers, sugar snap peas, mangetouts, mild chillies, peas, sliced avocado, baby asparagus, sliced mushrooms, artichoke hearts, olives, roasted vegetables.

Consider (if having salad as a main meal): A little cold cooked chicken or turkey (skinless), cold sliced duck or game (skinless), a few crispy bacon bits, lean cooked meats, Swiss cheeses (cubed, sliced or grated), feta cheese, goats' cheese, cottage cheese, cooked peeled prawns, flaked mackerel, faked hot-smoked salmon or trout, anchovies, sardines, fresh or tinned tuna, crab or salmon, sliced or chopped boiled egg or whole quail eggs.

To finish: Slug of extra virgin olive oil or nut/seed oil, lemon or lime juice, balsamic, red or white wine vinegar, sea salt flakes, ground black pepper, soya sauce, fresh nuts (whole, toasted, chopped or flaked), seeds, natural yoghurt or cottage cheese, wholegrain mustard, crushed garlic or ginger, drizzle of honey, spoonful of creamed horseradish, spoonful of peanut butter, tahini, houmous or tzatziki, shake of chilli or curry powder, Worcestershire sauce, Tabasco, tomato purée, sprinkling of chopped herbs.

If you are going for shop-bought salads:
Keep all of the above guidelines in mind, ensure that leafy greens and fresh vegetables form at least 50 per cent of the mix and if not, bulk it out with an extra bag of green leaves and as recommended for your lunchtime salad, bin the little packet of dressing that is often included and loaded with sugar and splash on your own using some of the following:-

— Extra virgin olive oil
— Linseed oil
— Nut and seed oils
— Avocado oil
— Lemon or lime juice
— Balsamic, red or white wine vinegar
— A dollop of houmous
— A dollop of cottage cheese or natural yoghurt
— A spoonful of wholegrain mustard or creamed horseradish
— A spoonful of nut butter
— Crushed garlic and/or grated fresh ginger
— And top with a few toasted nuts or seeds

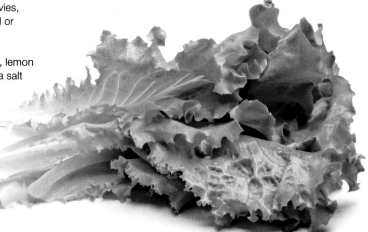

Healthy snacks

Great things to nibble when you get peckish...

- A couple of oatcakes with a slice of turkey and a slice of goats' cheese Cheddar
- One sesame seed Ryvita with almond butter and sliced tomato
- One slice of rye toast with mackerel pâté and slices of cucumber
- A small pot of natural yoghurt (Total 0% Greek) with a drizzle of honey and toasted flaked almonds
- A small pot of natural cottage cheese with chives
- V8 or carrot juice and a couple of oatcakes with nut butter
- A bowl of no-sugar muesli mix with nuts and seeds (no dried fruit) with soya/rice milk
- Pickled herrings with rye toast soldiers

- Small bowl of porridge with honey
- Soya milk latte
- Raw baby vegetables with houmous, tzatziki, natural yoghurt, cottage cheese, salsa or guacamole
- Small pack of raw unsalted nuts or nuts and seeds
- A couple of Ryvita with a chopped, boiled egg (mix in a little natural yoghurt and chopped fresh herbs)
- A couple of mini oatcakes with tinned salmon and cucumber slices
- A nut or nut/seed bar (no dried fruit)
- A couple of fresh celery sticks filled with nut butter
- A cold boiled egg and a couple of slices of cooked ham
- A cold cooked chicken leg/breast (skin removed), a couple of tomatoes and a small handful of fresh nuts
- A small pack of mixed olives with feta cheese cubes, or a small bowl of olives stuffed with anchovies or almonds
- Three-bean salad from the supermarket deli section
- Half an avocado stuffed with salsa and topped with chopped pine nuts
- A small tray of mixed fish and vegetable sushi
- A slice of toasted pumpernickel bread, spread with tzatziki and topped with thinly sliced smoked salmon and some cucumber or avocado slices

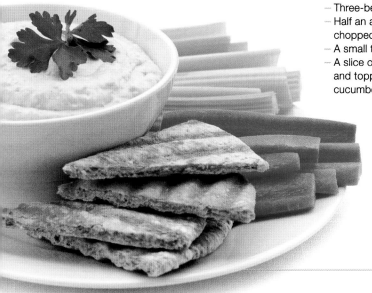

Seriously tasty dinners

Quick and easy meals in minutes

Beef stew

Prep and cook time: 30 mins

Ingredients: (for 2 servings)
1tbsp olive oil
1 small onion, finely sliced
½ garlic clove, finely sliced
150g beef stir-fry strips
½ yellow pepper, deseeded and thinly sliced
200g chopped tomatoes
Small sprig rosemary, chopped roughly
1 heaped tbsp pitted black olives

Method:
1 In a medium-sized saucepan, sauté the onion and garlic in oil until softened.
2 Add the beef, pepper, tomatoes and rosemary, bring to the boil, then turn down heat.
3 Simmer for 15 mins until the meat is cooked through, adding some boiling water if necessary.
4 Stir through the olives and serve.

Vegetarian alternative:
Leave out the meat and cook ½ chopped aubergine and ½ chopped courgette along with the pepper. Top with feta cheese cubes.

Turkey burgers

Prep and cook time: 25 mins

Ingredients: (for 2 servings)
250g turkey mince
Pinch dried thyme or 1tsp fresh
½ lemon
Sea salt and freshly ground black pepper

For the relish:
100g cooked peeled beetroot (not in vinegar), finely diced
½ small red onion, very finely chopped
1tbsp finely chopped parsley
1tsp olive oil
1tsp wholegrain mustard
Little gem lettuce to serve

Method:
1 Put the turkey mince into a bowl with the thyme.
2 Finely grate in the zest from the lemon and add a little seasoning.
3 Use your hands to mix the ingredients well, then shape into 2 equal patties.
4 Chill until ready to cook (can be frozen for up to 1 month).
5 Mix the beetroot with the juice from the lemon and the onion, parsley, oil and mustard.
6 Grill or barbecue the burgers for about 6 mins each side and serve with the beetroot relish and lettuce.

Spicy prawns

Prep and cook time: 20 mins

Ingredients: (for 2 servings)
1tsp olive oil
1 small onion, finely chopped
1tsp turmeric
2 garlic cloves, crushed
2cm piece ginger, grated
2tsp chilli flakes
400g tin chopped tomatoes
200g raw peeled prawns
1tbsp low fat yoghurt
Sprig fresh coriander, to serve

Method:
1 Sauté the onion in the oil until it starts to soften.
2 Add the turmeric, garlic, ginger and chilli and keep cooking for a few minutes until you end up with a rough, fragrant paste.
3 Add the tomatoes and simmer for 10 mins, adding a splash of water if you need to.
4 Stir in the prawns and cook until they turn pink.
5 Serve with a dollop of yoghurt and coriander.

Frittata

Prep and cook time: 40 mins

Ingredients: (for 2 servings)
3 eggs, lightly beaten
Pinch freshly grated nutmeg, plus a little extra
1tbsp olive oil
½ clove garlic, finely chopped
3 handfuls frozen peas, defrosted
75g buffalo ricotta cheese, broken into chunks
15g finely grated Parmesan
Rocket leaves, to serve

Method:
1 Season the beaten eggs with a little salt and freshly ground black pepper and the pinch of nutmeg.
2 Heat ½tbsp olive oil in a hot frying pan, add the eggs and leave to cook.
3 Add the remaining olive oil to another frying pan, add the garlic and peas and cook gently until cooked and any moisture has evaporated. Season to taste with salt and freshly ground black pepper.
4 Dot the pea mixture over the cooking eggs and add the ricotta. Adjust the seasoning again and grate some more nutmeg on top.
5 Cook for another 2-3 mins then scatter the Parmesan over the top.
6 Slide the frittata onto a large plate, then return it to the pan so that the uncooked side is now at the bottom. Cook for a further 5 mins, or until the frittata is set. Slide onto a plate and serve with rocket leaves on the side.

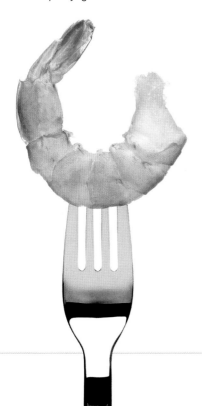

Beef stroganoff

Prep and cook time: 30 mins

Ingredients: (for 2 servings)
1tbsp oil
1 red onion, chopped
2 garlic cloves, chopped
1tsp paprika
1 green pepper, chopped
200g mushrooms, sliced
2tbsp red wine vinegar
150ml beef stock
200g lean rump steak, sliced and all fat removed
150ml 0% fat yoghurt

Method:

1 Heat the oil in a pan and fry the onion for a few minutes, until soft.
2 Add the garlic and paprika, and cook for 1-2 minutes until fragrant.
3 Add the pepper and mushrooms and fry for 5-8 minutes until softened.
4 Add the vinegar, boil to reduce until almost evaporated, then pour over the stock and bubble for a few minutes until thickened slightly.
5 Add the beef and cook for 2-3 minutes depending on how rare you like it. Then stir in the yoghurt (gradually to prevent splitting) and season.

Fish fillets Thai-style

Prep and cook time: 30 mins

Ingredients: (for 2 servings)
2 fish fillets, each weighing about 140g
A small piece of fresh root ginger, peeled and chopped
1 small garlic clove, chopped
1 small red chilli, deseeded and finely chopped
Grated zest and juice of 1 lime
1 baby bok choy, shredded
2tbsp soya sauce

Method:

1 Place the fish fillets on a banana leaf or large square of foil and scatter the ginger, garlic, chilli and lime zest over them.
2 Drizzle the lime juice on top and then scatter the pieces of bok choy around and on top of the fish.
3 Pour the soya sauce over the bok choy and loosely seal the banana leaf with string, or seal the foil, to make a package. Leave space at the top for steam to circulate as it cooks.
4 Steam for 15 minutes. (If you haven't got a steamer, put the parcel on a heatproof plate over a pan of gently simmering water, cover with a lid and steam).

Tomato, squash and spinach curry

Prep and cook time: 30 mins

Ingredients: (for 2 servings)
1tbsp olive oil
1 small onion, finely sliced
1tbsp Madras curry paste
½ small butternut squash, peeled and cut into small chunks
3 tomatoes, quartered
50g spinach leaves, roughly chopped
Sea salt and freshly ground black pepper

Method:

1 Sauté the onion in the oil until softened.
2 Add the curry paste and cook for a further 3 minutes.
3 Add the squash, tomatoes and 100ml water and stir well.
4 Cover and simmer for around 15 minutes until the squash is just cooked and the tomatoes have broken down.
5 Stir through the spinach and leave to wilt. Season to taste.

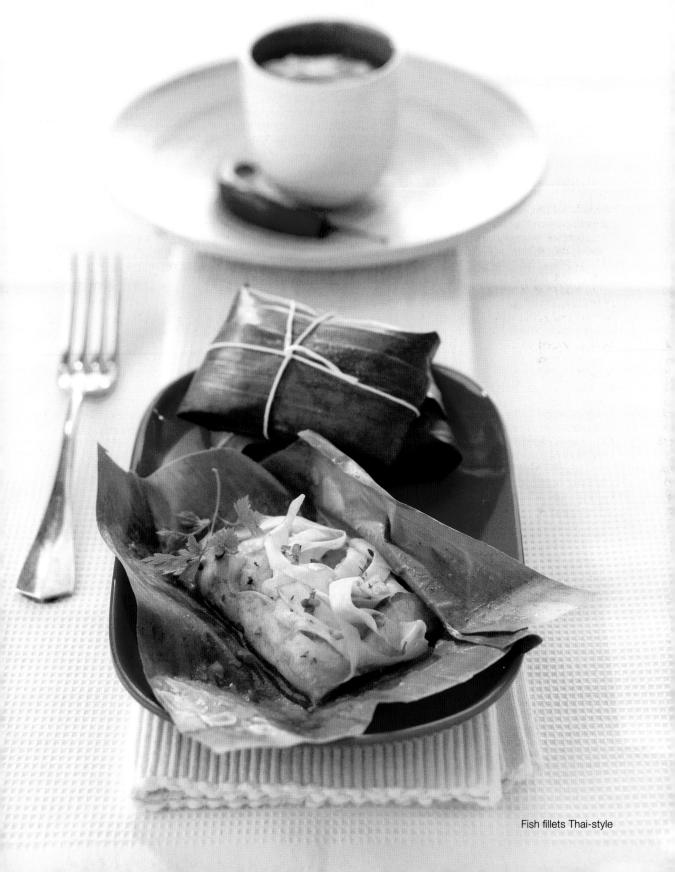

Fish fillets Thai-style

Super-quick and healthy dinners!

Very quick salmon

(serves 1) Lightly paint a salmon fillet or salmon steak with olive oil and grill under a moderate heat for 7-8 mins, turning once. Sprinkle with soya sauce, Worcestershire sauce or balsamic vinegar and lime or lemon juice just before serving.

Very quick chicken

(serves 1) Steam a skinless chicken breast either on a plate (cover it loosely with tinfoil/greaseproof paper) over a pot of simmering water or in a steam basket for 10-15 mins until cooked through. Spread pesto or black olive tapenade paste on top and put under the grill (low heat) for a couple of minutes until bubbling.

Very quick fish

(serves 1) Grill or microwave a couple of white fish fillets until fish flakes easily (4-6 mins dependent on type/thickness of fish). Warm through a couple of tablespoons of tomato salsa while the fish is cooking. Top the fish with the salsa and sprinkle with chopped herbs, freshly ground black pepper and lemon juice at the last minute.

Very quick omelette

(serves 1) Preheat the oven to 375F/190C/gas mark 5 and lightly grease a small baking dish with olive oil. Beat two eggs in a bowl and add anything you fancy from the fridge (see below for suggestions). Season with sea salt and pepper and pour into the prepared dish. Bake for 15-20 mins or until the top is slightly golden and a knife inserted in the middle comes out clean. Let it cool for a few minutes before serving.

Ingredients:
– diced cold ham
– diced cold cooked chicken
– diced Swiss cheese
– sweet peppers/artichokes/sun-dried tomatoes in jars
– freshly chopped parsley/basil
– whatever you have in stock!

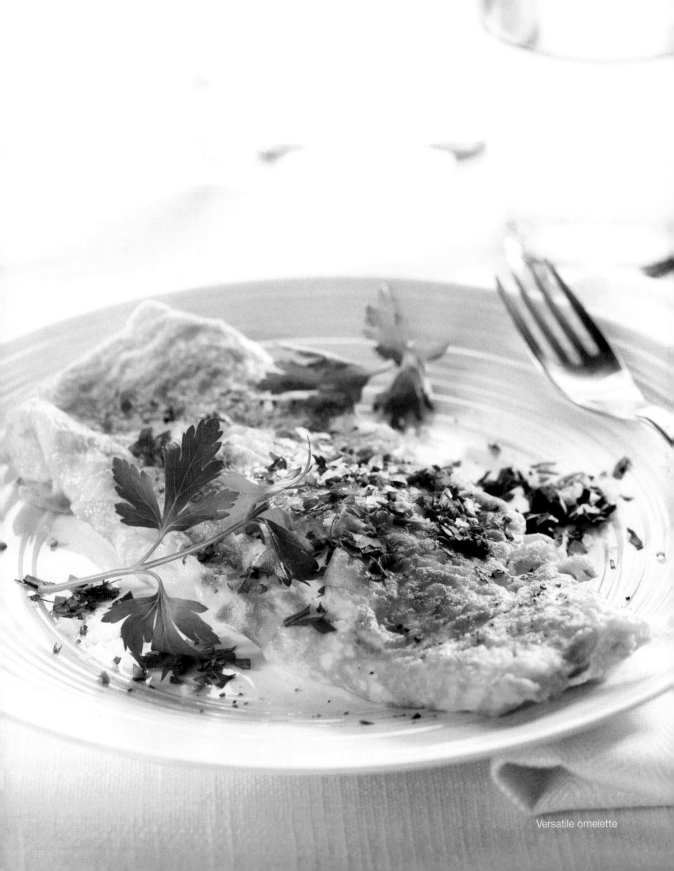

Versatile omelette

Very quick pork

(serves 1) Mix a spoonful of peanut butter with a little sweet chilli sauce and season with pepper. Put 2 thinly sliced pork fillets on a baking tray, brush the tops with half the nutty mixture and grill under a moderate heat for 2 mins. Carefully turn the pork over, brush the other side with the remaining mixture, then grill for another 2 mins or until just cooked through. Serve with fresh apple slices and chopped fresh coriander and/or mint.

Very quick lamb

(serves 1) Rub a lamb steak with a mix of lemon zest, a pinch of cinnamon and a splash of olive oil. Grill under a moderate heat for 4 mins each side if you like it pink, longer for well done. Put on a warm plate and leave to rest for a few minutes while you heat through a little fresh orange juice with very finely diced red chilli then pour this over the lamb.

Very quick prawns

(serves 1) Coat half a dozen fresh prawns with chilli, garlic or lemon-infused olive oil and grill both sides until pink but still succulent (2-6 mins depending on the size of the prawns).

Very quick mackerel

(serves 1) Bake a couple of smoked mackerel fillets (skin side down) in a medium hot oven, about 4-5 minutes.

Very quick burger

(serves 1) Use freshly ground lean beef or soya mince which has been soaked as per packet instructions. Add some sea salt crystals, ground black pepper and other spices of choice (cumin, coriander, curry powder, chilli powder etc), plus a few shakes of Worcestershire sauce or balsamic vinegar. Mould into burger shapes and chill for 15 mins before grilling. Top with a slice of goats' cheese Cheddar towards the end of cooking until melted and bubbling.

Very quick tofu

(serves 1) Cut firm tofu into cubes and stir-fry quickly in a little olive oil mixed with crushed garlic and grated fresh ginger. Add a squeeze of runny honey and top with toasted flaked almonds.

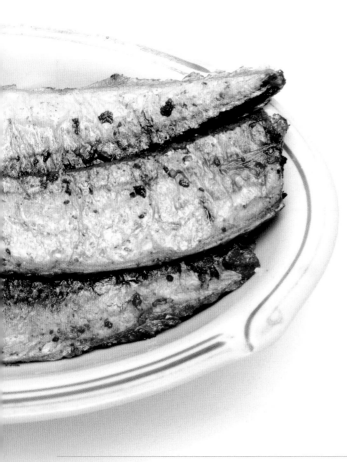

Go veggie

How to jazz up your vegetables and really boost their flavour

To get the maximum health boost from your veg, it's best to pick vegetables that are in their most natural state, and scrub them well or peel (if absolutely necessary). This way you know that you are getting lots of fat-burning fibre, vitamins and minerals plus a wealth of protective antioxidants.

If your life is a constant rush, however, go for frozen vegetables, as they retain many of the above properties; or ready-to-cook bags, which don't quite pack the same nutritional punch but still deliver lots of goodness.

If you're steaming or microwaving your veggies, make sure they retain their colour, still have a bit of bite and look enticing on the plate. Keep testing them with a sharp knife to ensure they don't overcook.

Roasting or baking them, if you have time, will bring out the deep flavours. Cut them into big chunks, coat lightly with olive oil, season with salt, pepper and finely chopped herbs and turn regularly (if some cook more quickly than others, just remove them while the others cook through and pop them back in for the last couple of minutes).

Or, grate or slice your veg finely and stir-fry it quickly in a teaspoon or two of olive oil for a tasty base to many dishes.

Make them even more delicious by adding some of the following towards the end of cooking or just before serving:

– A splash of vinegar
– A drizzle of honey
– A little marmalade or jam
– Toasted nuts and/or seeds
– Herb and spice mixes in olive oil
– A few drops of soya or fish sauce
– Finely chopped parsley, basil, mint or coriander
– A few finely chopped sun-dried tomatoes or grilled peppers and some of their oil
– A drizzle of nut or seed oil

Steam, grill, roast and get inventive with your veggies!

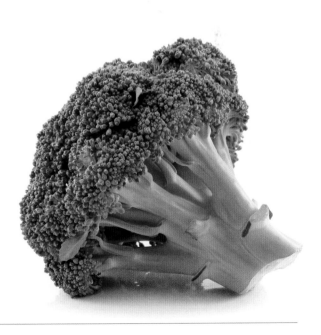

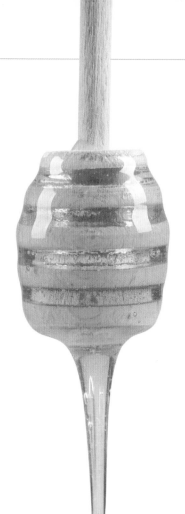

Tasty treats

For when you really fancy indulging

These won't do much damage as long as you regard them as treats and not as regulars during the 2-week diet. Only include when you are close to your fat loss goal (or if you are really struggling without sugar before then). Also, see The Quick Fix Rescue Plan for a few sweet treat choices that won't do too much harm.

– Muffins, waffles and pancakes – buy the wholegrain packet mixes and top with low fat soft cheese and sugar-free jam
– Dried fruit poached in tea
– Fresh fruit dipped in 70% dark melted chocolate
– Berry compotes (watch the sugar content)
– Halved peaches filled with crushed amaretti biscuits, drizzled with honey then grilled
– Fruit crumbles (use muesli mixes, a little butter and honey for topping)
– Plates of chopped, sliced and whole fruits with slices of cheese (ricotta, feta, Parmesan) drizzled with balsamic vinegar
– Dates filled with pecans, almonds or walnuts
– French toast topped with poached or fresh fruit
– Homemade or good quality bought carrot cake, banana cake or fruit loaf (lose the icing)

Stay hydrated

These are the healthiest drinks to sip

— Water, of course, but it can get a bit dull so opt for the sparkling version from time to time and add lots of ice, fresh strawberries, fresh lime, cucumber, fresh mint or a splash of fresh fruit cordial.

— Black, green, redbush or fruit/herbal teas without milk or sugar. Try them chilled on crushed ice, topped up with water and add a spoonful of honey and some fresh lemon or lime juice.

— Good quality coffee from ground beans with no milk or sugar. Do it the European way and have a large glass of water alongside. Have a soya latte or cappuccino with no sugar occasionally if you are feeling seriously deprived.

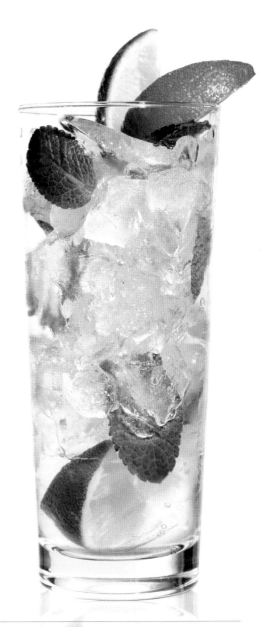

The quick-fix rescue plan

How to stay on track when you're always on the go

On-the-go heroes

Things can go horribly wrong for dieters when you haven't eaten for a few hours. Hunger strikes, you haven't planned ahead, and temptation lies at every turn. Many studies indicate that we tend to panic in mini supermarkets, service stations, airports, railway stations, corner shops or takeaways and we either make poor choices or eat nothing. Neither route helps fat loss, so rescue tactics are vital.

Regard this section of the book as an ally. Photocopy it from the book and keep it near you at all times – it will seriously limit potential damage. Some of the suggestions are not 100 per cent in tune with the 2-week diet in this book, but they will help you stay on track.

Sandwiches, wraps and baguettes

— Go for brown bread, rolls or baguettes, the denser the better and take the top off to form an open sandwich.
— If a single sandwich is on offer, grab it (half the damage of a two-pack).
— Pick the ones that are filled with salad or vegetables.
— Opt for fresh or tinned salmon, crab, tuna, beef, lamb, chicken or beans/chickpeas, so you get a decent amount of protein to fill you up quickly.
— If it looks creamy, there's likely to be too much mayonnaise, so avoid it if you can.
— If you prefer a wrap, unwrap it, grab a fork, eat the contents and bin most of the wrap.
— When you are in a pick-your-own fillings shop, get them to pile your selection into a box, ignore the roll and dig in.

Soups

— Thick soups are best when you are ravenous because they fill the void quickly.
— Soups with beans, lentils, chickpeas, peas, broad beans, sweet potato or butternut squash involved won't do anything like the damage of those packed with the white stuff (i.e. potato, pasta or rice).
— Asian-style soups are generally fine because they include fat-burning spices. Coconut milk is often involved, but is a better choice than cows' milk or cream because it is richer

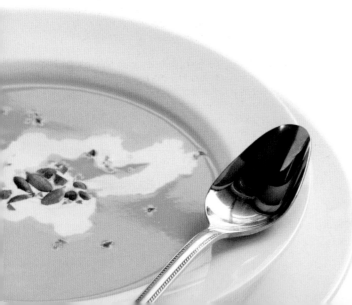

in healthy fats. Many are bulked up with noodles or rice, but if you sip the soup and leave the starchy carbohydrates at the bottom of the pot you won't go far wrong.
- If you opt for a vegetable soup, grab a small pack of fresh nuts or seeds to have on the side so you get some protein to make sure hunger doesn't return all too quickly.

Snacks

- **Raw unsalted nuts and seeds** are packed with filling protein and fat-burning good fats, so they can't be beaten when hunger strikes. But, to ensure you don't hoover a huge bag in one go, buy small packs, add a piece of fresh fruit and a small chunk of Cheddar cheese.
- **Salty snacks** deliver little other than quick but short-lived satisfaction, but if there is little else on offer you can limit the damage by opting for a small bag and scoffing a few slices of pre-packed ham, chicken or beef.
- **Cheese** can pile on the pounds if consumed regularly and in large amounts, but it can be a great hunger-buster if you make the right choices. Portioned and small packs are available everywhere. Go for hard cheeses, Swiss cheese, goats' cheese and ewes' milk cheese to reduce the saturated fat content. Better still, have a pot of cottage cheese (go for the ones with added extras or throw in a small pack of nuts and raisins if you are not a big cottage cheese fan).
- **Tinned fish** can be a bit messy and smelly, but salmon, sardines, anchovies, mackerel, crab or pilchards squashed onto a couple of Ryvitas will fill you up quickly.
- **Oats** are great when you are hungry. It's not hard to find a tub of ready-made porridge or a cereal bar rich in oats, and while many are laced with sugar, they are still a better choice than a burger and chips or a BLT. If you can get your hands on a packet of oatcakes, some houmous and a few baby tomatoes, so much the better.
- **Fruit** is a morning (and on its own) requirement on *The Ultimate 2-Week Fat Loss Diet,* but if there is little else available, no matter what time of day, grab it. Whether it's fresh, dried, with nuts, in a smoothie or yoghurt or in a salad mix, fruit is always going to be a better choice than a pasty or a slice made with fat-laden pastry.
- **Sweet treats** do little to nourish the body. So how do we satisfy our sweet tooth without straying too far from the fat-loss path? Small is beautiful – a kids' size bar of chocolate will deliver the sugar hit with less than half the sugar of a standard bar. And stay away from low-fat treats: often they have more sugar than the originals. Look out for the following when it's got to be sugar

- A bran muffin
- A few dates filled with pecans or almonds
- A fruit scone
- A kids' pack of chocolate buttons
- A pack of two shortbread fingers
- A small fruit yoghurt
- A small packet of wine gums
- Fruit, nut and seed bars
- Mini bar of dark chocolate (70% cocoa solids)
- Slice of banana loaf
- Slice of carrot cake (bin the icing)
- Slice of fruit cake (bin the icing)
- Small frozen yoghurt

Main dishes

- **Italian:** Selection of cold meats/cheeses, chicken or meatballs in tomato/pepper sauce, mixed fresh salads. Body swerve the pasta and potatoes, and if it *has* to be pizza, choose the thinnest base, go easy on the cheese and make sure it is stacked to the gunnels with heaps of vegetables and fish or chicken.
- **Indian:** Poppadoms with spicy onions, dhal, kebabs with yoghurt/cucumber sauce, tandoori chicken, lamb or beef with a little sweet/sour sauce on the side. Say no to the rice and naan bread.
- **Chinese:** Egg drop soup, hot and sour soup, prawns with ginger and spring onion, satay chicken, pork or beef, bean casseroles, stir-fried vegetables. Avoid anything with noodles or rice or leave them on the side.
- **French:** Onion soup (bin the cheesy crouton), soup Provençal (lots of vegetables in there), tuna Niçoise salad, coq au vin, moules marinières, beef bourguignon. Ask for extra vegetables/salad and don't have mash potatoes, Dauphinoise or frites.
- **Burger places:** Go for a plain burger, ketchup and mustard on the side won't hurt. No need for the bun or the fries, and get them to sling as much salad into the box as they can.
- **The kebab shop:** Not a great choice for fat loss, but if it's your only option refuse the pitta, ask them to put lots of salad in a box with grilled chicken and top it with the yoghurt dressing.
- **Pie and pasty shops:** Don't go there – find an alternative!

Other dangerous situations

In a bar: Ask for a bowl of olives and/or fresh nuts if they are available or go next door to the corner shop if there is one and grab a pack of oatcakes, cereal bar or a banana and munch it down quickly. Salty snacks on the bar are way too moreish when you are having a drink and you haven't eaten for a while. Even a bit of cheese will stem the need for these diet disruptors.

Room service: When you arrive at a hotel and you are tired and hungry, it's hard to stick with the programme if you haven't planned ahead and room service is your only option. Go for a steak, grilled chicken or fish with lots of vegetables or salad if you are there early enough, but if it's late the menu is often limited to a Caesar salad (bit too much mayo, but not a bad choice), a burger (ask for no bun, no fries and lots of salad), some sort of chicken and rice dish (ask for more chicken, sauce etc and lose the rice), a club sandwich (see if they might be willing to give you all the filling on top of just one slice of toast), or if you're lucky, a plain or filled omelette. No matter how poor the selection they always have salad to hand, so ask nicely and you can get lucky! There are also things the staff can be coerced into adding to the tray, like olives and nuts, which can help to satisfy your appetite. Always worth a try!

On a plane: If you haven't planned ahead and you are on a long-haul flight things can get tricky. Your best bet is to drink loads of water, get fresh and dried fruit and nut snacks whenever the trolley passes by and when the meals arrive, eat the protein and stay away from the bread, potatoes, crackers, biscuits and cakes. If it's a short flight have a tomato juice and a packet of fresh nuts, and if you are still hungry at the other end, grab a healthy snack at the airport so you are not hungry and tempted to gorge when you get to your final destination.

On the road: If you spend a lot of your day on motorways you are sorted, as many of them now have mini supermarkets where you can pick up some great healthy snacks to keep you going. But if you are restricted to service stations and roadside eateries, it gets a whole lot harder to keep up your fat-loss plan. However, you can usually get a breakfast anywhere at any time of the day. Ask for eggs (scrambled, boiled or poached, not fried), a couple of rashers of bacon (cut the fat off), grilled tomatoes and mushrooms and baked beans. Don't be coerced into the sausages, fried bread, black pudding and toast on the side. A healthier version of the Great British breakfast will keep you nourished for hours, and you need only top up with some fresh fruit and a packet of nuts later in the day and not too much damage will have been done.

Glossary of terms

Absorption: the process by which nutrients are taken from the intestines into the bloodstream, then into the cells.

Acidic: having a pH of less than 7.

Adrenaline: a hormone that is produced by the adrenal gland when stress or danger is sensed by the body. It increases blood pressure, heart rate and blood flow to muscles.

Aerobic: describes a bodily process using oxygen as a fuel.

Alkaline: having a pH of more than 7.

Amino acids: the basic building blocks from which proteins are assembled. There are eight essential amino acids, which must be derived from the protein foods we eat to enable the body to rebuild and repair.

Anaerobic: describes a bodily process not using oxygen as a fuel.

Antioxidants: dietary substances capable of neutralising free radicals that, in excess, could otherwise damage body tissue and lead to cell dysfunction.

Body mass index (BMI): a measure to estimate the ideal weight of a person based on their size and weight.

Basal metabolic rate (BMR): The rate at which the body converts food to energy, as measured at rest. It is taken 12 hours after eating, after a restful sleep, with no exercise, activity or emotional excitement preceding the test, and at a comfortable temperature.

Calorie: a unit used to measure the energy provided to the body by a food or drink. One calorie is defined as the amount of energy needed to raise one cubic centimetre of water by one degree centigrade.

Calorie: a unit used to measure the energy provided to the body by a food or drink. One calorie is defined as the amount of energy needed to raise one cubic centimetre of water by one degree centigrade.

Carcinogens: a substance capable of causing cancer in living tissue.

Cardiovascular: referring to the heart and blood vessels.

Cell membrane: the barrier that separates a body cell from its outside environment and controls what moves in and out of the cell.

Coenzyme: a non-protein compound that is necessary for the functioning of an enzyme. Many coenzymes are derived from vitamins.

Cofactor: a compound that is essential for the activity of an enzyme.

Detoxification: the process of getting rid of toxic matter from the body.

Diabetes: a chronic metabolic disease, characterised by abnormally high blood glucose (sugar) levels. It results from the inability of the body to produce or respond to the hormone, insulin.

Diuretic: an agent that increases the formation of urine by the kidneys, resulting in water loss.

DNA: the genetic coding found in the nucleus of every body cell which determines specific characteristics and functions within the body.

Electron: a stable atomic particle with a negative charge.

Enzymes: made up of a complex of amino acids, enzymes are part of every chemical reaction in living things. These include all digestive processes, growth and building of cells, any breakdown of substances such as vitamins and nutrients, and all reactions involving the transformation of energy.

Essential fatty acids: linoleic acid (omega-6) and linolenic acid (omega-3) are 'essential' because the body cannot work without them, but it cannot make them by itself, so they must be provided by food. They are important for brain development, controlling inflammation, blood clotting, heart health etc. Good sources include oily fish, nuts and seeds and olive oil.

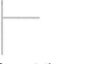

Fermentation: an anaerobic process that involves the breakdown of dietary components to yield energy.

Free radicals: highly reactive molecules possessing unpaired electrons that are produced during the metabolism of food and energy. They are believed to contribute to the molecular damage and death of vital body cells and may be a factor in ageing and disease. Antioxidants help to neutralise them.

Gene: a region of DNA that controls a specific hereditary characteristic, usually corresponding to a single protein.

Glucagon: a hormone responsible for helping maintain balanced blood sugar levels. When blood sugar levels get too low, glucagon activates glucose production in the liver, as well as regulating the release of glycogen from muscle cells.

Glucose: a six-carbon sugar which plays a major role in the generation of energy for living organisms.

Glycaemic index (GI): the blood glucose-raising potential of the carbohydrate in foods. The GI is calculated as the area under the blood glucose curve after a test food is eaten, divided by the corresponding area after a control food (glucose or white bread) is eaten. The value is multiplied by 100 to be a percentage of the control food.

Glycogen: a large chain of glucose molecules used to store energy in cells, especially muscle and liver cells.

Hormone: a chemical, released by a gland or a tissue, which affects or regulates the activity of specific cells or organs. Complex bodily functions, such as growth and sexual development, are regulated by hormones.

Immune system: the body's defence against infectious organisms and other invaders. Through a series of steps called the immune response, the immune system attacks organisms and substances that invade body systems and cause disease.

Insulin: a hormone secreted by the beta-cells of the pancreas, required for normal glucose metabolism.

Neurotransmitter: a chemical that is released from a nerve cell and results in the transmission of an impulse to another nerve cell or organ. Dopamine and serotonin are neurotransmitters.

Laxative: a food, compound or medication which, when consumed, either induces bowel movements or loosens the stool.

Macronutrient: nutrients required in relatively large amounts; namely carbohydrate, protein and fat.

Malabsorption: poor absorption of nutrients from food.

Metabolism: the sum of the processes (reactions) by which a substance is taken in and incorporated into the body or detoxified and excreted from the body.

Micronutrient: a nutrient required by the body in small amounts, such as vitamins and minerals.

Minerals: nutritionally important elements which are composed of one kind of atom. They are inorganic (do not contain carbon, unlike vitamins and other organic compounds, which do).

Monounsaturated fats: fatty acids with only one double bond between carbon atoms.

Neurotransmitter: a chemical that is released from a nerve cell and results in the transmission of an impulse to another nerve cell or organ. Dopamine and serotonin are neurotransmitters.

Pancreas: a small organ located behind the stomach and connected to the small intestine. The pancreas synthesises enzymes that help digest food in the small intestine and hormones, including insulin, that regulate the body's blood glucose levels.

Nutrient: any substance that can be metabolised by a living creature to provide energy and build tissue.

Omega-3 and **Omega-6:** linoleic acid (omega-6) and linolenic acid (omega-3) are essential because the body cannot work without them. For more, see 'essential fatty acids' on page 125.
Optimum health: in addition to freedom from disease, the ability of an individual to function physically and mentally at his/her best.
Oxidation: a chemical reaction that occurs when two substances interact, which removes electrons from an atom.
Oxidative damage: damage to cells caused by free radicals.

Pancreas: a small organ located behind the stomach and connected to the small intestine. The pancreas synthesises enzymes that help digest food in the small intestine and hormones, including insulin, that regulate the body's blood glucose levels.
pH: a measure of acidity and alkalinity.
Phytonutrients: compounds derived from plants in our diet.
Polyunsaturated fats: fatty acids with more than one double bond between carbon atoms.
Protein: a complex organic molecule composed of amino acids in a specific order. The order is determined by the sequence of nucleic acids in a gene coding for the protein. Proteins are required for the structure, function and regulation of body cells, tissues and organs and each protein has its own unique functions.

Satiety: refers to the feeling of satisfaction or 'fullness' produced by the consumption of food.
Saturated fats: fatty acids with no double bonds between carbon atoms.
Small intestine: the part of the digestive tract that extends from the stomach to the large intestine. The small intestine includes the duodenum (closest to the stomach), the jejunum and the ileum (closest to the large intestine).
Supplement: a nutrient or phytochemical supplied in addition to that which is obtained in the diet.

Thermogenic: descibes bodily processes that produce heat.
Thyroid: a butterfly-shaped gland found in the neck that secretes thyroid hormones. Thyroid hormones regulate a number of processes within the body, including growth, development, metabolism and reproductive function.

Vitamin: an organic (carbon-containing) compound necessary for normal bodily function. These compounds cannot be synthesised in adequate amounts by the body, and must therefore be obtained in the diet.

Small intestine: the part of the digestive tract that extends from the stomach to the large intestine. The small intestine includes the duodenum (closest to the stomach), the jejunum and the ileum (closest to the large intestine).

Index

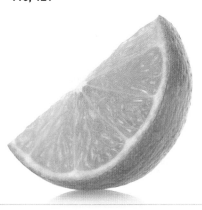

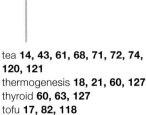

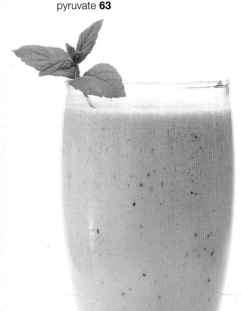